DECIPHERING THE SYSTEM

A Guide for Families of Young Children with Disabilities

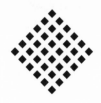

PAULA J. BECKMAN, GAYLE BECKMAN BOYES

BROOKLINE BOOKS

Copyright © 1993 by Brookline Books

Library of Congress Cataloging-in-Publication Data

Beckman, Paula J., 1952-
    Deciphering the system : a guide for families of young children with disabilities / paula J. Beckman and Gayle Beckman Boyes.
       p.   cm.
    Includes bibliographical references (p.   ) and index.
    1. Handicapped children--Services for--United States.
    2. Handicapped children--Education (Preschool)--United States.
    I. Boyes, Gail Beckman, 1955-   . II. Title.
    HV888.5.B4   1993
    362.4'048'083--dc20   92-7303
                                              CIP

Published by
Brookline Books
P.O. Box 1046, Cambridge, MA 02238-1046

Table of Contents

Dedication

We dedicate this book to three individuals who each, in their own way, taught us what it means to be part of a family.

To

Jacob Burdette Boyes
who inspired this book

To our mother,

Alberta A. Beckman
for her constant love and support

and

To the memory of our father,

Donald P. Beckman
whose integrety, strength and wisdom
remain a part of all of us who loved him

Acknowledgments

Many individuals have generously given of their time and their knowledge to make this book possible. We would like to thank Betty Pollins for the many hours she spent on various drafts; Abigail Herres, Rebecca Lee, and Linda Smith Myers for their contributions to the appendices; Carol Ann Baglin and Bobby Stettner-Eaton for their thoughtful reviews of various chapters; and all of the authors who contributed their time and expertise to this effort. We would also like to thank our husbands, Bob and Jim; our families, Victoria, Jon, Jacob and Julia; and Velma Buckner for the encouragement, love, and support they gave us as we completed the book.

Most importantly we would like to thank the many different families who reviewed the chapters and who contributed their time, ideas and experiences to this effort. We hope that we have passed on at least some small part of what they have taught us.

Preface

Ann Turnbull
Beach Center on Families and Disability
The University of Kansas

It strikes a chord with me that the authors, Paula Beckman and Gayle Boyes, are sisters with a shared family experience. Chapter 1 begins with Jacob's story. Jacob is Gayle's son and Paula's nephew. The significance of that is direct and strong: It reminds us that families consist of more than mothers. So frequently the field of disability studies has defined "family" to mean "mothers". As a result, we rarely get to hear the perspectives of fathers, aunts, uncles, grandparents, brothers and sisters, and other family members. Having a family team work together — a mom and aunt — provides the family dimension that is the cornerstone of this book.

The book begins by telling Jacob's story and grounding us in the reality of how one life can transform and strengthen a family. Jacob's story truly is the "Power of One" because he has impacted both his family and now all of us as readers, teaching us lessons already learned from his short life. Once again, this is an opportunity for us to affirm the positive contributions of children with a disability to our family and professional endeavors.

Deciphering the System presents a comprehensive, understandable, and relevant guide that gently and meaningfully provides families with all they need to know to be successful. Like a friend, Paula and Gayle will take you, the reader, by the hand and lead you through this complex process. They have a way of taking the frustration and confusion out of the process and even leaving you feeling as if you have just completed a conversation.

The chapters are replete with information about how families can help ensure that the educational program is genuinely geared to the preferences, strengths, and needs of their child and also of their family. There are hundreds of good ideas of how to act on rights and opportunities with many very concrete, step-by-step suggestions.

The final special feature of the book includes an excellent listing of national and state resources and also a comprehensive glossary of many of the specialized terms that are used in the field of disability. This resource material can be extremely helpful to families as they work to decipher the educational system.

I am reminded of the maxim:

Give a man a fish and feed him for a day,
Teach a man to fish and feed him for a lifetime.

I urge you to read this book carefully because it truly will teach you to "fish" in terms of accessing educational services; and consequently, it will "feed" you for a life time in terms of your own empowerment. Like Jacob, it is within you to be the "Power of One". One of your positive contributions can be deciphering the educational system for your own child and, thereby, transforming it for thousands of others.

CHAPTER 1

Introduction

Paula J. Beckman and Gayle Beckman Boyes

The news that a child has or is at risk for a developmental disability is often among the most frightening and confusing pieces of information that parents will ever receive. While everyone's experience is somewhat unique, we have found that parents also share many feelings.

As editors of this book, our experiences in this regard have been different. As a professional, Paula Beckman has worked with young children who have disabilities and their families for over fifteen years. Over the years she has seen and talked to dozens of families whose children have many different types of disabilities. As a mother of a young son with disabilities, Jacob, Gayle Boyes has first hand learned about the issues facing families of children with disabilities. She has lived in three different states and learned how many differences there can be between states in the way that services are provided. As sisters, we have shared our experiences and learned from each other. This book evolved because we realized that many families are looking for basic information so that they can understand and negotiate the service system.

JACOB'S STORY

At the time that Jacob was born, there were no apparent disabilities. With the exception of some external hemangiomas (you may have seen these relatively common "strawberries"), he seemed, in all ways, to be a healthy, normal infant. As he grew, Paula was concerned that his development seemed a little slow and everyone noticed that he did not always seem to see things. Although Jacob was seen several times by a pediatrician and an opthamologist, we were always told that he was fine. But there was always a lingering doubt about his development. Finally, he was seen by a pediatrician specializing in children with disabilities and our doubts were confirmed. During the many follow up visits to the neurologist and other specialists, it was determined that Jacob had a rare neurological disorder. He is legally blind (although he can see some things in part of his visual field), and has developed a seizure disorder. The doctors were not sure whether Jacob would survive.

When our family received this news about Jacob we were shaken in a way that eventually changed us all and continues to change us even now. As a family, we found bonds that were stronger than any of us realized and strengths that we never knew we had.

Although the details of Jacob's disability are complicated and relatively unique to his situation, the issues we faced as a family have been experienced by many families. The gut level knowledge that something was wrong, despite reassurances from his regular pediatrician, is only one example. Another experience, common to many families, is receiving a great deal of conflicting advice. Upon diagnosis, one physician wanted to do an emergency shunting procedure within two weeks; however, among the risks of the procedure were death, mental retardation and paralysis. When we finally found someone who could give a second opinion, we were told that there was no reason to shunt him, though he would have to be followed to monitor any neurological changes. As he has moved from state to state (and neurologist to neurologist) there have been no less than five different opinions regarding his neurological status. There have been different opinions from professionals on subjects as diverse as when to take his pacifier away, when and how to toilet train him, whether he needs vision services, and where he should be placed. In the end, it is always Gayle and her husband Jim who must make, and live with, the decision.

Like other families, we have experienced our share of competent professionals and our share of incompetent professionals; felt good about the services that Jacob was receiving, and felt that he was entitled to more; and met sensitive, caring professionals, and insensitive ones. We have waited for days for a phone call to be returned, traveled miles to appointments, and feared the reactions of other children.

As sisters, the challenges for us have been different. For Gayle, the challenges and the joys come daily. They involve gathering the strength for one more IEP meeting, wondering if and when and how devastating Jake's next seizure will be, watching him struggle with tasks that seem to come so easily to his sister, and learning how to make a complicated service system work to his advantage. They also involve watching the delight he takes when he succeeds at a task, his love of going to school, his amazing memory, and the gentleness he shows for his sister.

For Paula, the challenges are different. They involve frustration when a system that is supposed to work for children and families breaks down somewhere and anger when professionals who should know better are insensitive or condescending. However, there is also pride when the system works, when professionals go out of their way to make something happen and to make parents real partners. For our whole family, there is that incredible way that just a smile or a hug from Jacob can warm our hearts.

As parents and family members of a young child who has a disability, you undoubtedly share many of these and other emotions. In the midst of all of these emotions, one challenge that you will face is to understand the service system which has been designed for your child and family. It is a complicated system. At some point during your journey through this system, you are likely to experience both its best and its worst sides. At it's best, it provides a level of service to young children with disabilities which is historically unprecedented. At its worst, it can be complicated and confusing.

THE INFLUENCE
OF FAMILIES

During the past twenty to thirty years, the services available to children with disabilities have changed dramatically in the United States. These changes have brought increasing opportunities for children with disabilities. However, they did not come easily. They took the effort of many individuals who had a commitment to the rights of persons with disabilities and a vision of the type of services that should be provided. Many of these people were parents who brought court cases in behalf of their children and who lobbied politicians at all levels. Over and over, parents have demonstrated their power to influence the system and the importance of their role with respect to their children.

The evolution of services to younger and younger children is among the historic changes that have taken place. Gradually, the importance of services to young children was recognized, and over time the right to services have been extended from the school age population down to preschool. Indeed, infants are now receiving services in most states, although the nature and extent of these services vary somewhat on a state by state basis.

ABOUT THIS BOOK

Our purpose in putting together this book is to provide you with basic information about the early intervention and educational service delivery system. We hope that having this information will help you use the service system to your advantage. In talking to many parents, particularly parents of young children, we have found that many are unaware of how to best exercise their rights. Although most have had some information provided to them by their school or early intervention program, it is not always clear that the system can be used to work for them. For some parents, information about their rights may have been part of the "fine print" or buried in the midst of other information. For others, the information may have been provided during a difficult, emotionally charged period when many other decisions were being made. This book is intended to provide information about many aspects of the service delivery system which you may have questions about. It represents a joint effort between parents and service providers. In addition to the basic information that we have provided, we have also tried to address some of the feelings and concerns that we have heard expressed by families over the years.

In Chapter 2, *Entitlements and Rights: The Promise of the Individuals with Disabilities Education Act,* Florian and Greig provide a straightforward summary of those features of the Individual with Disabilities Education Act (IDEA) which are directly relevant to young children with disabilities and their families. The chapter includes information on federal eligibility requirements, the kinds of services that are required by federal law and basic information about how to exercise your rights.

In Chapter 3, *Dealing with Multiple Professionals,* Beckman and Kohl describe the types of professionals that you are most likely to encounter as you make your way through the service system. These authors also provide strategies for coping when you receive conflicting advice from different professionals and suggestions for interacting with different professionals.

Chapter 4, *Managing the Information,* offers ideas about how to handle the vast array of information you will receive as your child proceeds through the service system. It describes strategies for obtaining and collecting relevant information about your child's disability, as well as organizing the information, records and appointments that can quickly become overwhelming.

The focus of Chapter 5, *Educational Assessment,* is on basic information about your child's assessment. It includes information about the purposes of educational assessments that are done, the domains that are usually assessed in young children, and the types of assessments that are used. It also provides some ideas about how you can contribute to this process in order to provide the most accurate and useful information possible about your child.

Chapter 6, *Gathering Information About Families,* is designed to address the issues which arise when professionals seek information about your family. It describes the kind of information which may be sought, the reasons it may be needed by professionals, ways that you can make sure that your family's concerns are addressed, and strategies you can use to set limits if you feel that someone is being too intrusive.

Chapter 7, *The IEP/IFSP Meeting,* is focused on the meetings that are held to discuss the Individual Education Plan or the Individual Family Service Plan. In addition to explaining the purpose of these meetings and some of the general rules about how these meetings are supposed to be handled, we provide some strategies that you can use to make sure that your voice is heard and that you are truly an equal partner.

In Chapter 8, *Handling Transitions,* Fowler describes some of the issues that arise when your child must change programs. She describes the federal requirements about such transitions, and ways to prepare for these transitions.

Chapter 9, *Due Process,* is concerned with one of the most difficult exchanges that parents may encounter in their dealings with the early intervention or school system, the due process hearing. In this chapter, Edmister describes how to prepare for the hearing and how to present your case for maximum impact. She also gives some tips about how to handle yourself during and after the meeting.

In Chapter 10, *Opening Many, Many Doors,* Smith shares her personal experiences as a parent of a child with disabilities. She describes how she was helped through parent to parent support and ways that you might also access support from other parents.

At the back of the book you will find a glossary of terms that you may hear as you make your way through the system. There is also a list of state and national resources that are available to help you locate and access information specific to your state and to your child.

As family members of young children with disabilities, we all share many of the same hopes, fears and frustrations. Our circumstances are different and yet we share many common experiences. The vast majority of professionals are caring individuals who want to do a good job for children and families. As family members, there is much that you can teach, as well as learn, from the professionals you encounter. Your contributions are not just allowed, they are desperately needed.

To maximize your influence on this process, it is important that you are as informed as possible. You are far better off negotiating from a position in which you clearly understand your rights and are aware of the alternatives. This book is a first step in becoming so informed. It will provide you with a general idea about your rights under current Federal policies. It is important to follow this up by finding out specific information concerning your state's policies. You can obtain such information by contacting the lead agency in your state (if your child is two years of age or less) or your state education agency (if your child is three years of age or more). It is also important to be aware that refinements in the legislation and the corresponding regulations occur regularly. The information in this book reflects the most recent information available regarding the laws and regulations. However, you should always make sure you are acting on the most recent information. If you have questions, contact your state's lead agency or state education agency. Finally, it is important to integrate all this policy information with your special knowledge of your child.

We know the information provided in this book can help clarify some of the questions you may have. Just reading the material in this book is a positive step toward gaining knowledge and becoming an advocate for your child. As you gain more experience in dealing with the professionals and agencies serving your child, you will become increasingly knowledgeable and confident. You can be a powerful advocate for your child, a source of support for other parents, and make an important contribution to the system.

CHAPTER 2

Entitlements and Rights: The Promise of the Individuals with Disabilities Education Act

Lani Florian and Diane Greig

Introduction

Children with disabilities and their families have legal rights to early intervention and special education programs. These rights are granted and protected by federal law. The method by which the federal law is implemented in a state is through a state law that incorporates the requirements of the federal law. For this reason, the ways in which the requirements in the federal legislation are carried out may vary slightly from state to state. In general, the state law is more specific than the federal law. Sometimes it is more expansive. This chapter will familiarize you with the components of the federal law. It will provide you with information about the services your child and family are entitled to, and about your rights when it comes to obtaining those services. Although your state law may be slightly different, it will have been modeled on the components presented below. Strategies for using the rights granted under the law are also included.

No one knows a child like a parent. As a parent, you have a unique knowledge of your child's needs. Under the law, you have the opportunity to share this special knowledge with the professionals who serve your child. The importance of the parent's participation in the assessment process (chapter 5) and in the development of program plans (chapter 7) cannot be overestimated. A child's program, when developed in partnership with the parent(s) will always be superior to one that does not include the parent's knowledge of the child. This is the case regardless of the skill, competence, or prestige of the professional team. The parent brings context and perspective to the team.

To be your child's strongest advocate, it is important to be knowledgeable about the early intervention and special educational programs that serve your child and the laws that govern these programs. Federal law acknowledges the authority of the parent in decision-making by including sections which spell out the rights of parents. These sections, sometimes referred to as "due process", empower parents. Due process means fairness in decision-making. When due process protections are included in a law they are known as procedural safeguards. Procedural safeguards ensure that individual rights are protected and that people are treated fairly. If you are uncomfortable with the recommendations being made about your child, if you feel things go wrong in implementing you child's plan, you the parent can do something. Learning how procedural safeguards work will enable you to advocate on behalf of your child.

THE FEDERAL LAW

The federal law which authorizes early intervention and special education programs for infants and children with disabilities is called the Individuals with Disabilities Education Act (IDEA). Until recently, the law was known as the Education of the Handicapped Act (EHA) and many people still use this title. In 1990, the title of the law was changed and the term "handicapped" was replaced with the term "disability". The IDEA contains several Parts. Two Parts, Part B and Part H, authorize programs for infants and young children with disabilities and their families.

Part B of the IDEA was first created in 1975. It is widely known by its public law number, P.L. 94-142. This law requires states to provide "a free and appropriate public education" to all children, regardless of type or severity of disability. In other words, school-aged children can not be excluded from school because of a disabling condition. School-aged children are defined as children aged six to seventeen.

Originally, the federal law included incentives for states to go beyond serving school aged children with disabililties and provide services for children and youth with disabilities from age three through 21. Many states took advantage of these incentives by extending the right to a free and appropriate public education to three to five year olds (preschoolers) in the state law. As a result of the incentives and requirements of the federal law, the right to public education was secured for millions of children and youth with disabilities. In addition, thousands of children were able to receive early intervention and preschool programs. Despite this progress, access to services was not universal. Access depended on where a child lived, rather than what he or she needed. Many young children with disabilities still did not have the opportunity to receive services. A growing awareness of the fundamental unfairness of this situation helped pave the way for a new federal program which provides services for children with disabilities beginning at birth.

This occurred in 1986 when P.L. 99-457 added a new Part to the federal law. The new Part is called "Infants and Toddlers with Disabilities." It is Part H of the IDEA. Part H offers financial support to states that adopt state laws or policies that require early intervention services for infants and toddlers with disabilities and their families. The term "infants and toddlers" refers to children from birth through age two years, until the third birthday. Many of the requirements of Part H were modeled on the requirements of Part B, but there are differences. The differences reflect the needs of infants and toddlers with disabilities as compared to preschoolers and older children (ages 3-5 years). The basic components of the federal legislation in Part B (P.L. 94-142) and Part H (P.L. 99-457) are presented below.

State Administration. Under Part H (birth through two years), the governor appoints a "lead agency" responsible for coordinating and administering early intervention programs for children from birth through age two. Parents of children under the age of three should know the lead agency in their state. A list of lead agencies for all states is provided in the Appendix. For Part B (three to 21), the State Education Agency is responsible for administering the law.

Eligibility Definitions. The state must determine which infants and young children are eligible for services. Under Part H (birth through two years), infants and toddlers experiencing developmental delays, or those with a physical or mental condition likely to result in developmental delay, are eligible for early intervention services. A developmental delay is often first noticed by the parent when the child does not speak, play or get around as expected. Conditions that may result in a developmental delay may be genetic, the result of a hearing or vision problem, or may be due to damage to a baby during pregnancy, birth, or infancy. Some states provide services to children who are "at risk" for developmental delay. The specific definition of "at risk" is determined by the state. Examples of conditions that might place a child at risk for developmental delay include medical complications associated with prematurity, or problems associated with the child's environment, such as having parents experiencing psychological problems. Under Part B (three to 21), children who have conditions such as mental retardation, autism emotional disturbance or learning disabilities; as well as those with vision, hearing, speech, orthopedic, or other health impairments are eligible for services. Preschoolers (children aged three through five years) experiencing a developmental delay are also eligible for services. It is possible that a child who is eligible for services under Part H (birth through two years) will not be eligible for services under Part B. Eligibility under Part B is more limited than Part H. For example, in some states an infant born before term may be served under Part H whether or not the infant demonstrates a developmental delay. This is because preterm infants are at risk for later developmental problems. Under Part B, the same child would only be eligible for services if he or she were identified under one of the disability categories contained in the law.

Developmental Services for Infants and Young Children with Disabilities. Both Part H (birth through two years) and Part B (three to 21 years) require that services be provided based on a written plan designed specifically for an individual child. Under both Parts, the services required are based on the child's specific needs.

Part H (birth through two years) requires early intervention services for infants and toddlers with disabilities, and their families. The law states that early intervention services may include: family training, counseling, and home visits; special instruction; speech pathology and audiology; occupational therapy; physical therapy; psychological services; service coordination services; medical services for diagnosis and evaluation; early identification, screening, and assessment services; and health services that will enable a child to benefit from early intervention services; vision services; assistive technology devices and assistive technology services; and transportation and related costs that are necessary to enable an infant or toddler and the infant or toddler's family to receive early intervention services.

As you can see, early intervention includes a range of services. These services must be provided by qualified persons. Generally this means the person should have a degree, license, or certificate that qualifies him or her to provide a specific service.

Under Part H (birth through two), early intervention must be provided in natural environments. The child's home or day care center is an example of a natural environment. A natural environment might best be determined by asking where the child might be if not for the need for early intervention. If he or she would otherwise be at home, or in day care with siblings or peers, then the home or the day care center would be the natural environment.

Part B (three to 21 years) requires "special education and related services" for all eligible children. Special education is specially designed instruction. Related services are supportive services that enable a child to benefit from special education. These include: transportation; speech pathology and audiology; psychological services; physical and occupational therapy; recreation; early identification and assessment; counseling, medical services for diagnostic and evaluation purposes; school health services; school social work services; and parent counseling and training.

Special education and related services must be provided by qualified persons in the **least restrictive environment**. **Least restrictive environment** means that some or all of the child's education should take place with peers who do not have disabilities. The decision about placement in the least restrictive environment is made separately for each child based on the child's unique needs. What is least restrictive for one child may or may not be least restrictive for another child even though the two children may have the same disability.

Evaluation. Individual needs are determined through an evaluation process. Both Part H (birth through two years) and Part B (three to 21 years) call for comprehensive evaluation conducted by a multidisciplinary team. A multidisciplinary team brings professionals from several relevant disciplines together with the parent to participate in the evaluation. **Parental consent must be obtained prior to the evaluation.** Under Part B, the evaluation must be completed within 30 calendar days after the child is referred. Under Part H the evaluation must be completed within a 45 day time period. Generally, the evaluation includes an assessment by each team member. Assessment is discussed in detail in Chapter 5.

Written Plan of Services. After the multidisciplinary evaluation has been completed, a meeting which includes the parents as participants develops the educational or service plan. In the aftermath a written plan is developed. Under Part H (birth through two years), the plan is called an Individualized Family Services Plan (IFSP). Under Part B (three to 21 years), it is called an Individualized Education Plan (IEP). Both plans are prepared by a multidisciplinary team, which includes the parent. The IFSP and the IEP contain information from the evaluation such as present levels of development or educational attainment, goals and objectives that the child will be expected to achieve within one year, the services required to meet the goals, timelines and criteria for measuring progress toward these goals, starting dates and length of services, and who will provide them.

Part H (birth through two years) also requires a statement of the family's resources, priorities and concerns relevant to enhancing the child's development, the name of a case manager or service coordinator responsible for service coordination, and steps that will be followed during the transition of the child at the age of three from early intervention services to preschool.

The IDEA states that the IFSP and the IEP must be developed "within a reasonable time" after assessment. Although the state determines what is reasonable, it should not take more than 45 days from the time of referral to the initiation of services. In general, services are initiated after the plan is developed and the parents agrees by signing the written plan. With parental consent, services for children under the age of three may begin before the plan is completed. Once a plan is developed it must be reviewed to update it. The IEP must be reviewed yearly, and the IFSP is reviewed every six months. The parent can request more frequent reviews. Parents of children who received services under Part H (birth through two years) can request that the school use the IFSP instead of the IEP as the written plan of services during the preschool years.

Procedural Safeguards. Both Part B (three to 21 years) and Part H (birth through two years) of the IDEA contain provisions which grant parents certain rights. Although service providers and school districts are required to inform parents of their rights under the law, this does not always occur as intended. In 1989, both a Harris Poll and the National Council on Disability reported that parents frequently are not aware of their rights. Few professionals take the time to be certain that parents of children with disabilities understand their rights. The following section provides detailed information on the procedural safeguards which protect the right to early intervention and special education for young children with disabilities and their families. Additional information can be found in the chapter by Edmister.

PARENTS' RIGHTS

The idea of procedures to protect individual rights and assure fairness in decision-making is difficult for many parents and professionals to think about because no one expects to be treated unfairly. The human service professionals parents encounter are people who have chosen to work on behalf of children. When everyone has the best interest of the child at heart, it is difficult to imagine the necessity of procedural safeguards. However, they are necessary because no system is perfect.

Procedural safeguards protect children from the failures of the system. By including procedural safeguards in a law, policymakers build accountability into the system. Procedural safeguards are part of a system of checks and balances. The Part H (birth through two years) procedural safeguards are very similar to those in Part B (three to 21 years). Each of the general components is discussed below. Part B has some additional requirements which are noted.

Confidentiality. Under both programs, the privacy of the family is protected. This means that when an agency or school collects "personally identifiable information", such as information about the family, the child's disability, results of the multidisciplinary evaluation, assessments, and individualized program plans, it is available only to certain people, such as the child's teacher. This information may not be shared with others without parental consent. The agency or school providing services to your child has a list of persons who have access to personally identifiable information. One person is in charge of maintaining confidential records.

Examination of Records. The parent has access to all information in the child's file. Not only may the parent review the information, he or she can ask for a copy and an explanation of the information. The agency or school cannot refuse a parent's request to examine records, but, there may be rules governing how parents gain access to records. For example, the agency or school may require that someone be present while the record is being examined, that an appointment be made in advance, or that the request be put in writing. Even if this is the case, the agency or school must allow the parent to review the requested information within 45 days of the request.

Generally it is not difficult for parents to obtain access to confidential records. In fact, you have probably already received written information about what is contained in your child's record, and the rules about confidentiality and access. Usually this information is mailed to the home or given in the form of a handout at a meeting. Parents often think of this type of information as "the small print" and may not save or recall it. The important thing to remember is that you are **entitled** to the information. There may be rules about how to gain access to the information, but **the request to examine records cannot be refused**.

It is possible the parent may feel the information contained in the record is inaccurate. When the you disagree with the information contained in the record, there are procedures to follow so the information can be changed. The person with overall responsibility for confidentiality of records will be able to explain these procedures.

Under Part B (three to 21 years) there is an additional procedural safeguard which enables the parents to request an independent evaluation at public expense if they are in disagreement with the evaluation conducted by the school.

Written Prior Notice. Parents must be informed in writing before any changes can be made in the services their child receives. A change in services includes new evaluations of the child, changes in the child's early intervention or educational program, or the child's diagnosis. The written notice must be in the parent's native language.

The law requires that parents be informed of their rights. As stated earlier, experience has shown that efforts to comply with this mandate have not been satisfactory. Parents are often not aware that they have received information about their rights because it comes in a packet with a great deal of other information or because it is part of the "fine print" in the child's record. Further, the language used to inform parents of their rights often includes legal jargon.

Surrogate Parents. When the parents or guardian of a child are not known, not available or the child is a ward of the state, the state may assign what is known as a *surrogate parent*. The purpose of assigning a surrogate parent is to be sure that the rights of the child are protected. A *surrogate parent* is a person who serves as an advocate for the child, but who is not otherwise involved with the child. Such a person must have the knowledge and skills needed to be an advocate for the child. The surrogate parent has all of the rights of the natural parent when advocating on behalf of the child.

Timely Administrative Resolution of Complaints. You have the right to present a complaint about a child's identification, evaluation or placement. The specific procedures for making a complaint vary from state to state and they become more formal as the child enters the school years. Under Part H (birth through two years), the hearing for the administrative resolution of a complaint must be held at a time and place that is convenient for the parent and it must be concluded within 30 calendar days after the receipt of the parent's complaint. A parent who wishes to have a complaint heard must make a written request for a hearing. Hearings are helpful in situations where communication between the family and the professional team members has broken down, and attempts to solve the impasse through less formal channels have not been successful. However, hearings can be expensive because either side may bring an attorney to represent them.

Civil Action. Under both programs, the parent may appeal a decision to the courts (civil action). At this point, the parent should obtain legal advice if he or she has not already done so. Many parent organizations keep lists of attorneys who specialize in special education or disability issues. A good resource to contact is the Protection and Advocacy Organization in your state. The phone number is available through your governor's office, or you can contact the national office. The address and telephone number are listed at the end of the chapter. Under Part B (three to 21 years), but not Part H (birth through two years), the procedures include the recovery of attorney's fees if the court rules in the parent's favor.

Stay Put Clause. Services to a child cannot be disrupted during the time that a complaint is being resolved. The child should continue to receive services in the current placement. The placement can be changed only with the agreement of the child's parents and professional team.

EXERCISING YOUR RIGHTS

Specific due process protections vary depending on the age of the child. If your child is under the age of three, he or she is protected by Part H (birth through two years) of IDEA. After age three, a new determination of eligibility for services under IDEA must be made. A parent should not assume that a child who is eligible for services under Part H will automatically be eligible for services under Part B (three to 21 years).

Due process procedures may vary according to state law. As noted earlier, each state fulfills the requirements of the federal law through a state law incorporating the elements of the federal law. The procedures and policies for each state may be different.

Although the law under the IDEA grants rights to parents and their children, it is often not easy for parents to find out how to exercise these rights. If you are concerned about your child's development and would like to find out if he or she is eligible for services, or if you are unhappy with the services your child is receiving, the following suggestions may be helpful:

1. If you need information about services, state law and policies, or ways you can advocate on behalf of your child: National organizations that have information on the resources in each state are the National Information Center for Children and Youth with Disabilities (NICHCY), the National Association of Protection and Advocacy Systems (NAPAS), or the Technical Assistance for Parent Programs (TAPP). Addresses and telephone numbers for these organizations are listed at the end of this chapter.

Another source of information is the central directory maintained in each state which includes early intervention services, resources, and experts in the state. The directory may also include parent support groups and advocacy organizations. Professionals you have had contact with such as your child's pediatrician, day care providor, or teacher may be able to tell you how to get a copy of the central directory. The state Child Find office, the Governor's office, the lead agency for Part H, or the State Education Department will also have this information.

2. If you want to determine whether your child is eligible for services: Call the Child Find office or program in your state. The mission of Child Find is to locate and evaluate children with disabilities who are eligible for services. Parents or professionals may refer the child to Child Find to determine her or his eligibility for services.

3. If you are dissatisfied with the services your child is receiving: When you are in disagreement with the results of an evaluation consider an independent evaluation. An independent evaluation is conducted by professionals who are not employed by the lead agency or school district. For children served under Part B (three to 21 years), the costs of an independent evaluation are covered, but under Part H (birth through three years), the evaluation may be at the parent's expense. For disputes that you are unable to resolve with the service provider, *request mediation, if it is available.* Although some states provide mediation, it is not mandated in the federal law. Mediation is a way of resolving disputes without filing a formal request for an administrative hearing. It is a less adversarial, less formal, less costly means of resolving disputes. It generally involves bringing in an impartial third party to facilitate problem-solving when professionals and parents are at an impasse. It does not preclude or replace an administrative proceeding or civil action. It is a means of avoiding litigation in settling disputes.

If mediation is unsuccessful, *file a request for a formal hearing.* File the complaint with the lead agency if your child is under three years, or with the State Education Agency if your child is three years or older.

After you contact the appropriate agency, you will be informed of the specific procedures to follow in your state. In most states you will have to submit your complaint in writing, usually by filling out a form provided by the agency. Once the agency receives the complaint, it must respond to and resolve the dispute within 30 calendar days under Part H (birth through three years) and 45 days under Part B (three to 21 years). There is a longer timeline under Part B to allow for an administrative appeal at the state level if the hearing was held by a local school district. Furthur information about how to handle a due process hearing is presented in chapter 9.

BARRIERS TO EXERCISING YOUR RIGHTS

Despite the promise of the rights granted in the IDEA and the power of due process, problems exist. Many parents report feelings of intimidation when it comes to actually participating in the educational or service planning meeting. They may go along with a professional recommendation even if they disagree because they believe the professional knows more about the child's needs than they do. The parent may not want to "make waves" by disagreeing with the team.

Parents sometimes feel intimidated when it comes to exercising their rights. They are concerned they will alienate the professionals serving their children. They are worried about the cost of due process procedures. Many parents cannot afford legal representation even though in some situations they may be able to recover their costs if they prevail in a dispute. Parents believe they do not have an equal chance to win an argument because they perceive the professionals to be better equipped to present a case. For these reasons, parents often conclude that using the procedural safeguards is not in the best interest of their children. It is not known how many parents would use due process if these problems were eliminated. We do know that of all the children served, very few cases become the subject of an administrative hearing or court case. Some people use this as evidence that the system is working. Others say that the procedural safeguards themselves are not strong enough to assure fairness. It is hard to know which point of view is correct.

No parent enters the service delivery system with the expectation that they may or will need the support of due process procedures to obtain appropriate services for their child. Parents do not think: "I will sue for help." In fact, even when parents are aware of the procedural safeguards available to them, they often hesitate to use them. Parents frequently perceive them as costly, complicated, time consuming, risky and adversarial. Yet the due process safeguards provided in the law is the fundamental mechanism by which parents are empowered to fulfill their opportunity to participate in the decisions made for their child.

ADDITIONAL RESOURCES

The aim of this chapter has been to provide information about the federal law which establishes the right to early intervention and preschool services for young children with disabilities and their families. To this end, we reviewed the basic components of Part B (for children three to 21 years) and Part H (birth through two years) of the "Individuals with Disabilities Education Act" (IDEA). Children have been receiving services under Part B since 1978. Part H was established in 1986. At this time, most states are still developing service delivery systems for Part H. Although the goal of Part H is universal access to service delivery, there is much work that needs to be done before this is truly achieved.

In closing, we wish to note that both Part H (birth through two years) and Part B (three to 21 years) contain additional components that have not been covered by this discussion. These components pertain to a state's administration of the programs and do not directly affect the provision of services to children and their families. For further information about the legislation, or for a copy of the law and its accompanying regulations, contact one of the organizations listed below.

Additional organizations are identified in the Appendix.

It is also inportant to remember that from time to time there may be amendments to the law or changes in regulations. These organizations should be able to provide the most current information about such changes.

National Information Center for Children and Youth with Disabilities
(NICHCY)
P.O. Box 1492
Washington, D.C. 20013
1-800-999-5599

Technical Assistance for Parent Programs
(TAPP)
95 Berkley Street
Suite 104
Boston, MA 02116
617-482-2915

National Association of Protection & Advocacy Systems
(NAPAS)
900 2nd Street, N.E.
Suite 211
Washington, D.C. 20002
202-408-9514

REFERENCES

Harris, L. and Associates. (1987). *International Center for the Disabled Survey III: A report card on special education.* New York: Author.
Individuals with Disabilities Education Act. 20 U.S.C. 1400 et. seq.
National Council on Disability (1989). *The education of students with disabilities: where do we stand?* Washington, DC: U.S. Government Printing Office.

CHAPTER 3

Working with Multiple Service Providers

Paula J. Beckman and Frances L. Kohl

One of the most common experiences that parents of young children with disabilities encounter is that there is a vast array of professionals who become involved with their child and family. One reason for this phenomenon is that it is unlikely that any one individual can address all concerns about a particular child. The extent to which your child and family are involved with more than one service provider will depend on the nature of your child's needs and on your family's priorities and concerns. In some ways it may be reassuring to know that there is a variety of resources available to assist you. On the other hand, the sheer number of persons with whom you must interact can be time consuming and confusing. In this chapter we will describe federal laws concerning the multiple services that your child may receive, the types of educational and early intervention teams that you may encounter, the advantages and disadvantages of receiving services from multiple providers, and issues you may experience encountering multiple service providers.

FEDERAL POLICIES
CONCERNING AVAILABLE SERVICES

The services your child receives differ depending on whether he or she is receiving services under Part H (birth through age two) or Part B (three and older). More information is provided about eligibility under these parts in Chapter 2. The policies differ with respect to the involvement of various service providers in two major ways. The first is whether your child must qualify for special education to receive other services; the second involves the specific services to which your child is entitled.

Services Available Under Part H

If your child is served under Part H (birth through age two), the law states that your child is eligible for **early intervention services**. Accordingly, early intervention services are services designed to meet the developmental needs of each eligible child under this part and the needs of the family related to enhancing the child's development. While these services can include special instruction, many other types of services are also included. An important distinction between Part H and Part B is that under Part H, children do not have to be eligible for special education to receive other types of services. These services must be selected in collaboration with parents, provided by qualified personnel, and be specified in the Individual Family Service Plan (IFSP).

There are many different early intervention services which qualify under Part H. These include (but are not limited to) audiology; service coordination (sometimes referred to as case management); family training, counseling and home visits; health services (which are necessary to enable a child to benefit from other early intervention services which he/she is receiving at that time; see pages 11 and 12 of this chapter for more information about which health services qualify); medical services (only for diagnostic or evaluation purposes); nursing services; nutrition services; occupational therapy; physical therapy; psychological services; social work services; special instruction; speech-language pathology; transportation services; vision services; and assistive technology services and assistive technology devices. Parents may decline any one of these services without jeopardizing access to other services.

Services Available Under Part B

If your child is three years of age or more, federal law provides that he is eligible for special education and related services. **Special education** is considered "specially designed instruction that meets the students unique needs, including classroom instruction, physical education, home instruction, and instruction in hospitals and institutions" (Turnbull & Turnbull, 1990). **Related services** are those services which the child needs to benefit from special education. Eligibility for such services is based on the results of evaluations by qualified personnel in a particular area. The decision that your child is eligible for related services is formally made at the meeting to discuss the Individual Education Plan (IEP) along with specifics regarding which services will be provided and the frequency and intensity with which these services will be provided. Once agreed upon in the IEP, the school system cannot make changes without holding another IEP meeting. Moreover, once the need for specific related services is identified on the IEP, those services must be provided even if they are not available within the school system. Often this is done by contracting with private individuals, other programs, or agencies. In any event, these services must be provided at no cost to you. The related services which may be provided include early identification and assessment, physical therapy, occupational therapy, speech pathology, audiology, psychological services, social work services, counseling services (including rehabilitation counseling), diagnostic medical services, school health services, counseling and training for parents, recreation (including therapeutic recreation), assistive technonogy services and transportation. However, this list of services is not exhaustive and other services can be identified on the IEP. According to Turnbull and Turnbull (1990), there are several factors that distinguish services which are technically considered related services from those that are not. Specifically the distinctions are: "a) the complexity of the service, b) the cost of providing it, c) the expertise required to provide it, d) the risk of liability for the provider (school) and of damage to the student if the service is not correctly provided, and e) the constancy or frequency with which the service must be provided" (Turnbull & Turnbull, 1990, pp. 220).

TEAM MODELS

The delivery of multiple services to young children with disabilities is accomplished in many ways. Three approaches or models have emerged, although there are overlapping features. These include multidisciplinary, interdisciplinary, and transdisciplinary models of intervention. These models differ according to the following components: (a) assessment, (b) the development of education and intervention plans (i.e., IEP's, IFSP's), (c) implementation, and (d) the method and frequency of communication and interaction among professionals and parents.

In the multidisciplinary approach, each specialist acts independently of their colleagues. Each specialist evaluates the child independently, makes recommendations for treatment without consultation with other specialists and provides services independently. Typically, communication is informal and inconsistent between professionals and parents.

In the *Interdisciplinary* approach, services are provided by each specialist though information is shared with team members. Like the multidisciplinary approach, each specialist evaluates the child independently, but team members share their assessment results and discuss treatment plans at team meetings. Specific treatment techniques are conducted by each specialist. Team meetings are conducted as needed or on a regular basis.

In the *Transdisciplinary* approach, most services are provided by a designated team member who along with other team members are responsible for sharing information and techniques and working together across disciplines. Team members (including parents) work together to gather information on each child's background, conduct observations, and implement discipline related assessments to acquire sufficient information to generate treatment goals. Team professionals and parents develop a service plan together based upon input from all team members. A primary service provider (PSP) is assigned who is responsible for assuring a coordinated and consistent treatment program. Team members assist and consult with the PSP in providing consistent treatment. Team meetings are held frequently to exchange information, instructional techniques, and outcomes.

Both the multidisciplinary and interdisciplinary models rely on a direct, traditional therapeutic approach to provide services (i.e., services are provided independently by each specialist). Although direct therapy has advantages, there are some disadvantages as well. Traditional, direct therapy has the following disadvantages:

- children are removed from the classroom and the teacher cannot view the therapeutic techniques and progress of the child;
- therapy is conducted in isolated areas devoid of normal distractions and typical interactions with others;
- treatment is provided only two or three times per week for a short period of time, making the gains minimal and difficult to transfer to other activities;
- there is limited information exchanged between professionals

and parents which may mean that the services may not be reinforced as well between sessions.

In contrast, members of a transdisciplinary team are responsible for sharing information across disciplines. Associated with the transdisciplinary model is the practice of **integrated therapy**. An integrated approach focuses on communication among parents, teachers, and therapists at all stages of service delivery: assessment, planning, implementation, and evaluation, thereby making a transdisciplinary model preferred by many professionals in the field (Raver, 1991). Together the team members observe and assess the child in natural settings to determine motor, communication, social, and cognitive areas of functioning. **Arena assessment** is encouraged and consists of one team member testing while others observe. As Raver (1991) states:

> Before an arena assessment, team members meet and identify behaviors they would like to see for their individual evaluations. Following the assessment, if the professionals in the arena did not observe all they needed, parent report items are used or another assessment time is arranged. Professionals who use arena assessment report it saves time, and that with training they can see what they need for their discipline-specific evaluations while also seeing the whole child (p. 34).

After an arena assessment, a joint determination is made by parents, teachers, and all related service providers on appropriate intervention goals. Goals are delineated and then prioritized based on input from the individuals who have daily and/or professional contact with the child. Although direct therapy is provided by the therapist, the concept of role release or **role sharing** is encouraged. *Role release* refers to a sharing and exchange of certain discipline-specific roles and responsibilities across team members (Lyons & Lyons, 1980). For example, the classroom teacher, who is with the child throughout the day, will learn from the physical therapist the appropriate positions and movements to be done with the child throughout the day. Since it is impossible for the physical therapist to be with the child every time the child must be repositioned, the teacher learns the necessary skills and provides the child consistent therapeutic skills which enhance learning throughout the school day.

In order to have a successful transdisciplinary team, members must be committed to working together and communicating with each other on a consistent basis. Members must learn to respect personal differences and characteristics, educational/discipline backgrounds and terminology, and treatment techniques and style. They all must share the common goal of providing the best services to young children with disabilities.

Advantages and Disadvantages of Dealing with Multiple Service Providers

To some extent, the composition of your child's team depends on the size and location of the program. In large systems, it may be more common to see larger teams. For example, in a large system, there may be a wide variety of professionals including a special educator, a physical therapist, an occupational therapist, speech/language specialist, a psychologist, and a hearing and/or vision teacher. Other professionals may also be part of your child's team depending on the needs of your child and your family. In contrast, smaller systems typically have smaller teams consisting of two or three primary disciplines obtaining consultation from other personnel or agencies as needed. For example, in a small system your child's team may include a teacher and a physical therapist with consultation from a speech/language specialist and a health professional.

There are advantages and disadvantages to each of these situations. On a larger team, there is a wider variety of disciplines represented and a wider range of expertise available. However, many parents feel intimidated by the sheer number of professionals who are present during meetings. There is also more opportunity for differences of opinion to be generated and to be presented with conflicting advice. With a smaller team, the parent may have a better opportunity to get to know and work with individual team members. IEP or IFSP meetings may seem less intimidating. On the other hand, if your child's disability is uncommon and/or his needs are very unique, it may be more complicated to obtain the special advice and assistance you need on the smaller team.

Professional Qualifications

When considering the variety of services to which young children with disabilities are entitled under federal law, it is easy to become confused about what types of professionals are able to provide a specific service. As Hanson and Lynch (1989) have noted, educationally oriented early intervention programs require individuals with a wide range of expertise. To obtain services, programs may look for individuals who have expertise in more than one area or have the same individual fill multiple roles.

In evaluating the expertise of the individuals providing services for your child, Hanson and Lynch (1989) note that it is important that they have the necessary certifications, licensures, or registrations required by your state and by their discipline. Hanson and Lynch (1989) believe that although this does not guarantee expertise, it provides basic assurance that they have received certain academic preparation, practical experience, and knowledge in their profession. These authors also point out that the experience and skill of specific professionals do not always correspond exactly to their preparation in a specific discipline. For example, a teacher or therapist may have excellent credentials in their discipline but have worked primarily with adolescents or adults and know very little about the development of infants and young children. It may help you to look past the specific discipline and find out if the individual has expertise working with children of the same age as your child. Keep in mind that even within the birth to five range, the needs of children are quite different: that is, infants have different needs than a child who is four or five. Also, do they have experience working with the special needs of your child? For example, while some pediatricians have experience treating the spacial medical concerns that children with Down Syndrome experience, others do not.

Special Services Under Part H

It is beyond the scope of this chapter to define and explain each of the individual disciplines and services identified under the law. Descriptions of most common disciplines serving the needs of young children with disabilities are provided in the glossary. For additional information on a specific discipline, you can contact the professional organization associated with that discipline. Many of those organizations are identified in the Resource List provided at the end of this book. Despite this caveat, we feel that it is important to describe at least two specific services because they are new in early intervention and there may be some confusion about which services are included under the law.

Service coordinator. One of the important distinctions between Part H (birth through age two) and Part B (three to twenty one) is that Part H requires the involvement of an individual known as a *service coordinator* (sometimes called a case manager). Your *service coordinator* is responsible for making sure that your child and family have access to the rights, procedural safeguards, and services which are authorized in your state. Every child and family who participates under Part H must be provided with this service. The service coordinator is responsible for helping parents gain access to the services identified on the IFSP, coordinating services across agencies, and making sure that services are delivered in a timely fashion. Service coordinators should perform a variety of functions. For example they should help coordinate the performance of assessments and evaluations; participate in the development of the IFSP; help identify available service providers; make sure that families know about advocacy services; and, when the time comes, help develop a transition plan.

Health services. While Part H limits health services to those that are necessary to enable the child to benefit from other early intervention services (during the time that they are receiving these services), certain services must be included for infants and toddlers because they are believed to meet the following criteria. According to the regulations, these services include:

> "(1) such services as clean intermittent catheterization, tracheotomy care, tube feeding, the changing of dressings or ostomy collection bags, and other health services; and
>
> (2) consultation by physicians and other service providers concerning the special health care needs of eligible children that will need to be addressed in the course of providing other early intervention services." (Federal Register, 1989)

However, certain services are not included in the regulations. These are services that are surgical in nature (such as cleft palate surgery), purely medical in nature, devices necessary to treat a medical condition, and medical-health services (such as routine immunizations).

SERVICE DELIVERY OPTIONS

The type of services that your child receives will depend upon the nature and severity of her disability, her age, and the particular service models that are being implemented in your area. You may encounter several different options.

Home-Based Services

Home based programs are most frequently offered for infants and toddlers. In a home-based program, the service providers come to your home at a specified time. For example, a teacher or developmental specialist may visit your home. Although there is variation with respect to the frequency of the visits, they typically occur once every week or two weeks. Other professionals (e.g., nurses, therapists) may also make home visits. Services are generally provided in your presence and the provider will probably want you to be included in the session. If you are working, the service provider may visit when the babysitter is present or may visit your child's day care facility. There are many advantages to home-based programs.

1. home-based programs give you the opportunity to interact directly with your child's service provider on a regular basis. As a result, you may find it easier to have your questions addressed and may feel more comfortable with individual members of your child's team.

2. You may also find that your child is more comfortable at home than in an unfamiliar environment such as a clinic. This is important because young children often behave differently when they are in different settings. The service provider has the opportunity to see how your child functions at home and may be better able to understand the questions you raise and the how to structure the treatment so you can support it in your home.

3. Home-based programs also have the advantage of occurring in the most natural environment possible for infants.

4. Finally, since the service provider visits you, you don't have to go through the process of getting your child ready to go out. This is especially nice during cold or wet weather when you may not wish to go out.

However, there are some disadvantages to home-based settings. First, because team members are not always present at the same time, coordinating the efforts of different team members can sometimes be more difficult. However, your team probably has developed some strategies to deal with this issue, so you should not let it discourage you from trying home visits if they are an option. Second, in most home-based programs, your child does not have as many opportunities to interact with other children. This may not be important to you if your child is very young. However, it may be quite important if your child is a little older and has limited opportunities to play with other children.

Finally, if your child must be seen by many different professionals, you may grow tired of the sheer number of individuals who are in and out of your house.

Center-Based Programs

If your child is in a center-based program, she will be brought to the center to receive services. In some programs, particularly center-based infant and toddler programs, parents are encouraged to participate as well. The major advantage of a center-based program is that they offer opportunities for contact with other children. They also provide some structure and routine. This will help your child prepare for the demands of more intensive preschool and kindergarten classrooms. The disadvantages include less flexibility in scheduling and little opportunity for the interventionist to observe how your child does at home. In addition, (depending on if and how the program involves parents) there tends to be less opportunity for direct, regular contact with interventionists than there is in a home-based program.

Integrated Programs

Integrated programs are center-based programs, which include children with and without disabilities. It is usually preferred that the program be a part of the larger community, rather than isolated. Thus, it is preferable to have an integrated preschool or kindergarten program within the context of a regular elementary school. There are many reasons that integrated programming is considered to be a best practice. First, there is no reason that any child should be isolated from other children simply because he has a disability. Second, there is evidence that children with out disabilities can benefit from being around children with disabilities, particularly if there are special efforts made to facilitate their interaction (Odom & McEvoy, 1988).

The nature and degree of integration depends on a number of factors. One factor is age. A younger child may be integrated in a day care center whereas a five year old may be integrated into a kindergarten classroom. Type of activity is also a factor; children may be integrated during some activities but not during others.

If you are considering enrolling your child in an integrated placement, several steps may help to promote a positive outcome.

1. Make sure that your child will receive any supports that he needs to function in the integrated placement. This may include simple environmental modifications such as moving him to the front of the class, or providing him with special equipment.

2. Encourage the regular program to prepare your child's peers. For example, the teacher (or you) might introduce your child to the class and explain that he can't see well or is unable to walk. Peers can be given little games to help them understand what it feels not to be able to do these things. Peers can also be given ideas about how they can help your child, how to play with him, what he likes to do, and how to communicate with him.

3. You and the other team members should decide whether your child will need other special supportive services. (e.g., a classroom aide, consultation from the physical therapist).

4. Visit the classroom occasionally to find out how things are going. Watch your child as he interacts with other children, observe whether he participates well in class activities. Talk to the teacher or developmental specialist about how the arrangement is working and what you can do to facilitate it.

ISSUES THAT MAY ARISE
WITH MULTIPLE SERVICE PROVIDERS

Federal policy clearly intends that parents should have an important and participatory role on the team. As parents, you frequently have information and suggestions that are critical to developing the most effective plan for your child and your family. However, as parents, it is often difficult to assume that role. Several issues can arise. The purpose of this section is to alert you to these issues and provide some suggestions for handling them.

Limited contact with service providers

Service providers often work with each other in many different circumstances and may know each other well. They may have well established routines with which you are not familiar. Because they are often interacting with one another frequently throughout the day or week, they have informal opportunities to discuss professional matters. As a parent, you may find it difficult to feel comfortable with a group that seems to know each other so well. While it is unlikely that you will come to know service providers in the same way that they know one another, there are ways to make yourself better acquainted so that you feel more comfortable.

The extent to which this is a problem for you will depend in part on the type of services you are receiving. It is also likely to differ from service provider to service provider depending on the needs of your child and family.

For example, if your infant or toddler is receiving home-based intervention services, you may find that you know the individual(s) providing this service well. In such instances, a teacher or other service provider may visit your home on a regular basis. Because you see this individual regularly, you have many opportunities to discuss your child's achievements, exchange stories, discuss needs that you and your family may face, ask questions, and generally communicate informally.

There is less opportunity for these discussions if your child receives services in a school or center-based program. In such instances, it may help to observe or volunteer in your child's program. You may want to visit when you know a particular specialist will be present so you have the opportunity to observe, ask questions, and develop a positive relationship.

Dominance of one member

You may find that one (or more) member of the team seems to dominate the discussions about your child. This may make for a difficult situation if you disagree with that team member or if you are unable to hear the views of others. One reason for the dominance of one individual may be simply due to personality differences. Another may reflect a kind of professional elitism as one member may view his or her discipline as more important or more critical to the needs of your particular child and family.

Regardless of the idiosyncracies, aggressiveness or the number and type of degrees an individual service provider has, you — the parent — are the ultimate decision-maker for your child. Your experience with your child, daily observations, interactions, and investment in your child's future are critical to the decision making process. For this reason, it is important that you receive input from the full range of individuals who are working with your child and family.

Before a meeting involving a dominant individual, think through your priorities and concerns for your child and family and prepare a written list. The list may help you focus your thoughts, on items important to you. If you have thought about important issues in advance, you will have some sense of what your spcific concerns are, the ways they are addressed, and whether and where to compromise if differences emerge.

You can also try several techniques to minimize dominance and reduce tension. First, assume an attitude that is positive and even-tempered. Then, listen quietly while the individual gives his/her opinion fully. Sometimes, people tend to state their opinion quite strongly or repeat it several times because they don't believe they have been understood. If you listen carefully, you may be able to alleviate this fear. It may also be helpful to restate what the person has said. For example, you may say something like, "So, if I've understood you correctly, you think that Sarah needs less isolated physical therapy because the teacher can do these activities in the classroom?" Once you have allowed the individual to fully state his or her case, it is appropriate to push for more balance in the conversation. For example, if the individual persists, you might say, "I think I understand your position, but I'm not clear about how Ms. Adams feels. I wonder if she could tell us what she thinks." By remaining calm but persistent, you may be able to achieve a somewhat more balanced perspective, and meet the needs you have addressed as important to your child.

Conflicting recommendations from service providers

As you begin to work with an increasingly large number of professionals, you may receive conflicting recommendations from different service providers. Conflicting advice can be extremely frustrating and confusing because it is often difficult to know whose recommendation to follow. This can be frightening if you are facing a serious medical crisis or facing critical placement decisions.

It is critical to recognize that honest differences of opinion among good professionals are not uncommon. Unfortunately, there are not always definitive answers. Professionals usually make their best judgment based upon their training and experience. However, differences can arise for several reasons. There may be different philosophical beliefs about the best course of action that should be taken in a particular circumstance. If service providers who disagree come from different disciplines, some of the differences may be rooted in their disciplinary training. For example, a teacher may focus on your child's cognitive skills whereas a physical therapist may focus on your child's motor skills. The recommendations they make often reflect these differences in focus. If conflicting recommendations are made, it may be because each professional has been trained to concentrate on a specific aspect of development. Even professionals from the same discipline may have different recommendations which result from seeing your child in different circumstances, differing experiences with other children, or holding different treatment and intervention philosophies.

At the outset, it is important to decide how critical the difference of opinion is. For example, if there is a difference of opinion about your child's next placement, you may consider it important and worth pursuing. Other differences may seem less important. For example, two professionals may have different ideas about when and how to begin spoon feeding. In this case, you are probably best advised to look at how the recommendations match your family's routines and your child's needs.

If you decide that it is important to resolve the difference, several strategies may be helpful. One strategy is to ask each service provider to give you more information about how they arrived at their recommendation. Once you know the basis for their recommendation, it may be easier to make a decision. For example, one service provider may have extensive experience with children who have disabilities that are similar to your child's whereas the other individual has very limited experience. Or you may find that one of the professionals has extensive experience working with specific professionals or in a specific program which she is recommending. She may know that the individuals in that program are particularly well-trained or experienced. Knowledge about the basis upon which each service provider reached his or her conclusions can help you make a more well-informed decision.

Another strategy is to ask other parents if they have had a similar experience. Input from other parents is often meaningful because they may share many of your feelings and concerns. Because other parents have "been there", they can often bring an entirely different perspective to your decision-making process.

It is also possible to obtain another opinion. If a third service provider agrees with one of the others, it may help you come to a resolution. It is also possible that a third individual may provide a solution that satisfies the concerns of everyone. However, obtaining a third opinion takes time and could cost money. It is also possible that the third service provider will offer a different opinion which may confuse matters further.

Another alternative is to ask for a meeting between yourself and the professionals who are giving you differing opinions. By bringing everyone together, you may be able to clarify why the recommendations are so different and encourage everyone to share their perspectives. It may be that the differences are not as pronounced as originally believed. It may also be possible to arrive at a compromise that addresses the issues which are the basis of the disagreement.

In some cases, particularly with interventions you are carrying out at home, you frequently have to try both recommendations to determine what works best with your child and in your family. For example, two professionals may recommend completely different approaches to some aspect of behavior management. The effectiveness of an approach may depend as much on specific characteristics of your child and your family's routines as it does on the specific merits of the approach. Don't be afraid to consider such recommendations in light of your own circumstances. Share those circumstances with the professionals with whom you are working so that they can help you adopt or adapt their suggestions.

Other issues

There may be differences of opinion about issues which are not related to your child and family as well as "turf" issues that you are not aware of. In some cases, these issues of disciplines may be the result of how the system is structured. Moreover, there may be individual personality or professional differences between individuals which existed before the difference of opinion over your child.

It is obviously not your role to resolve these kinds of differences. If you sense that the difference of opinion over your child is rooted in turf or personality issues, it is important not to allow yourself to become involved in them. Try to collect objective information about your alternatives. Think the issues through carefully and try to make your decision objectively, keeping your concerns and priorities foremost in your mind. If the problem persists, it may help to be straightforward and simply point out that the issues seem to go beyond your child and family. If they remain unresolved, you may need to request a change in service providers to minimize the effects on your child and your family.

SUMMARY

The wide array of providers who participate in services to young children with disabilities offer you a wealth of information and resources. At the same time, the sheer number of professionals also present challenges. As a general rule, you are most likely to overcome these challenges and maximize your chances of obtaining the most effective services for your child by doing the following. First, recognize your value. Second, do your homework (e.g., know your rights). Third, know your own priorities. And finally, don't be intimidated. You know your child better than anyone else and the decisions that are made will affect your entire family.

REFERENCES

Hanson, M. J. & Lynch, E. W. (1989). *Early intervention: Implementing child and family services for infants and toddlers who are at-risk or disabled.* Austin, TX: ProEd.

Lyon, S., & Lyon, G. (1980). Team functioning and staff development. A role-release approach to providing integrated educational services for severely handicapped students. *Journal of the Association for the Severely Handicapped, 5,* 250-263.

Odom, S. L. & McEvoy, M. A. (1988). Integration of young children with handicaps and normally developing children. In S.L. Odom & M.B. Karnes (Eds.), *Early intervention for infants and children with handicaps: An empirical base.* (pp. 241 - 268) Baltimore, MD.: Paul H. Brookes Publishing Company.

Orelove, F.P., & Sobsey, D. (1991). *Educating children with multiple disabilities: A transdisciplinary approach.* Baltimore, MD: Paul H. Brookes Publishing Co.

Raver, S.A. (1991). Transdisciplinary approach to infant and toddler intervention. In *Strategies for Teaching At-Risk and Handicapped Infants and Toddlers: A Transdisciplinary Approach,* (pp. 26-44). New York: Macmillan Publishing Company.

Woodruff, G., & McGonigel, M.J. (1988). Early intervention team approaches: The transdisciplinary model. In J.B. Jordan, J.J. Gallagher, P.L. Hutinger, & M.B. Karnes (Eds.), *Early childhood special education: Birth to three,* p.166. Reston, VA: Council for Exceptional Children.

CHAPTER 4

Managing the Information

Paula J. Beckman, Gayle Beckman Boyes, and Abigail Herres

In the days and months following your child's diagnosis, you will begin to collect a great deal of information from medical professionals, infant specialists, special education teachers, therapists, and possibly social workers or a service coordinator. This may be especially true if your child has multiple disabilities or when you must deal with multiple service agencies (for example, both the educational system and the health system). Even within one service system, there are often several professionals who provide services for your child. For example, if your child is seen in an infant or preschool intervention program provided by the school system, a team of professionals will probably see your child. These may include a teacher, a physical therapist, an occupational therapist, and\or a speech therapist. You may receive individual reports from each of the professionals who are involved with your child. These reports may be simple notes updating you on your child's progress, more formal reports of assessment results, and/or copies of the individual education plan (I.E.P.) or the individual family service plan (I.F.S.P.) which has been developed for your child and family. In addition, there are often reports from medical specialists, hospital records, insurance information and so forth.

As a result, you are likely to accumulate vast amounts of paperwork. This paperwork can be of enormous value as time goes on. Some of the information may be needed later if your child sees a new doctor or therapist or changes schools. You may need other records to document that your child needs additional services or to obtain insurance reimbursements. Some documents give you a record of your child's progress over time. Knowledge of how your child is progressing assists in program planning for your child and your family. In addition, such information may help establish the need for further services and be generally informative to professionals who are trying to assist you with your child's program. To make life easier for yourself, you may want to develop a system to help you manage all of the paperwork you must handle. By developing such a system you can be certain of finding the records you need when you need them. You will also have the necessary documentation for reimbursement from insurance and\or Medicaid.

GENERAL RULES ABOUT SETTING UP A SYSTEM

There are two major rules of thumb to keep in mind when organizing your system for keeping track of information about your child. First, *keep it simple*. Remember that the purpose of the system is to *reduce* the day-to-day hassles that sometimes come with making certain your child's needs are met. Any system which is too complicated or time-consuming will be more likely to *increase* than to minimize such hassles.

Second, create a system which is flexible. Your child's needs are likely to change a great deal as she gets older. Try to establish a system which can be adapted easily as your child's needs change.

BASIC COMPONENTS OF YOUR SYSTEM

In our experience, we have found six components in a system that can be great time-savers and reduce day-to-day hassles. You may have additional ideas that are useful to you. On the other hand, you may feel that one or more of these components is not helpful. If so, by all means, eliminate it.

Calendar

The time required to attend an early intervention program, to go to school and\or see multiple specialists can rapidly grow! You may find that you are constantly setting up appointments and making sure you get your child to them. Without a system for keeping track of all of these appointments, the situation can soon feel out of control. We have found that the most effective solution is to get (or make) *one* calendar on which you keep track of all your child's appointments. Keep it in a place where you can see it easily (on the refrigerator, near the telephone) and refer to it when you are scheduling appointments. Take it with you when you go to appointments which may require another visit.

Table 4-1
Basic Components of Your System

- CALENDAR
- TELEPHONE LOG
- PORTABLE FILE SYSTEM
- SUMMARY OF DEVELOPMENTAL MILESTONES
- COMMUNICATION NOTEBOOK
- CRISIS PLAN

Telephone Log

Have a place where you can note whom you have spoken to on the telephone, their telephone number, who placed the call, when you spoke to them, and what was said. Keep track of calls that you place, even if you don't actually have the opportunity to speak to the person. If someone calls you or if you speak to an assistant or a secretary, write down their name. If needed, such a log can provide a record of your efforts to obtain services for your child. It will also help if you need to relay information to a spouse or to another professional.

Some people may find it is helpful to keep the log on their calendar. This is a matter of preference, but has the advantage of providing clear information regarding dates when contacts with service providers were made.

In addition, in the front of your phone log, it is often helpful to keep telephone numbers of professionals that serve your child as well as pertinent information that you may need while on the telephone (examples: policy numbers from health insurance policies, patient account numbers, etc).

File System

You will need a place in which you can keep and organize your child's records. The system does not need to be complicated or expensive. However, you will probably find it most useful if it is portable so that you can take it to meetings and appointments with you. This can be as simple has having a box in which you always put letters, and records regarding your child. Our family has found it helpful to keep an old briefcase which has separate file folders for correspondence with the school (individual education plans, assessment reports and so forth), as well as files for insurance papers, medical records, and so forth. This system is convenient because it can be easily taken to appointments. When seeing a new medical specialist, copies of records can be provided immediately (sometimes avoiding a follow-up appointment). It is also possible to easily review last year's educational or service plan to see if goals have been met, or to document the recommendations of another professional. If copies are needed, they can be provided right away. This allows you to avoid the time lag involved when the new professional must seek your permission to obtain copies and wait for them to arrive.

There are many different way to set up your system. The system you choose will depend on how complicated your child's needs are, the number of professionals and agencies you see, and your own personal preferences. Ideas for such a system vary from having a notebook with different pockets; file folders; a shoe box in which everything is kept; or a box, crate or briefcase in which you keep different files or envelopes. Just put all of the correspondence, records, bills, and other materials together. To whatever extent possible, keep similar or related information together. As a general rule, there are two types of information you will want to collect: medical/health information and school information.

Medical/Health Information. Certain kinds of medical information will be necessary for the school as well as for other service providers.

- Schools often need a birth certificate as well as proof of immunizations in order to enroll the child in school.

- You will have to provide at least some medical information to a number of different professionals. This may include information about your family's health (examples: history of diabetes or heart disease), information about your pregnancy (examples: was your child full term, were there medical complications, at birth, etc), and specific details about your child (e.g., allergies, immunizations, childhood diseases such as chicken pox and measles).

- Be sure to keep a list of your child's doctors and their telephone numbers — the pediatrician as well as any specialists.

- Keep the name, address and policy number(s) for any health insurance providers you may have.

- Keep copies of the reports from various hospitals, doctors, and clinics as well as the reports you receive from various therapists.

- Keep copies of bills that you receive so that you can submit them to your insurance provider if your doctor's office or hospital does not submit them for you.

- You should also have information about medications (name and dosages) your child must take. It may help if you have this written down so that you can refer to it if necessary.

- One time-saver is to write such information down or make a copy of a form you filled out previously. You can then take copies to your appointments. The professional may be willing to refer to your copy rather than make you answer the same set of questions yet another time.

- Depending on the nature of your child's disability, it may be useful to request copies of relevant medical records such as MRIs and CAT scans. Although you will probably have to pay for these copies, such records can be extremely valuable if your child has a medical emergency which requires treatment by a physician who is unfamiliar with his or her case.

Such records may also be valuable, when obtaining a second medical opinion, in a move, or when changing physicians. Some parents report that they have encountered resistance when asking for medical records. If this happens, try not to become upset or feel intimidated. Remember that you have the right to see this information.

Program/School Information. Keep a file which includes information regarding your child's intervention program for each year. It is helpful to keep information about the program in which your child is seen (including the address and phone number), names of the program director or principal, teachers, therapists, and other personnel who are in contact with your child. This is also the place to keep copies of school records.

Remember, as a parent, you have a right to see and have copies of your child's records if you wish. This includes assessment reports, individual education plans, individual family service plans, the reports of specialists and so on. You can request that the program provide you with a list of the types of records that they are keeping about your child, where they are kept, how to see them. Keep in mind that the school may have different records in several different places, so it is probably a good idea to ask for this list. It is important to check these records to make certain that the information which is being kept is accurate. You also have the right to obtain copies of these records although you may be charged a fee for duplication. However, the fee cannot keep you from reviewing the records.

- A sample letter requesting information is provided at the end of this chapter.

- If you can't pay for the copies you need, tell this to school officials and the records should be provided for free.

- The records should be provided within a reasonable time frame (generally no more than 45 days).

- If the information is requested before an IEP meeting or before a due process hearing, the school is required to let you see the records before the meeting.

- If you feel that your child's records are inaccurate or do not reflect important information, you can request that they be changed. A sample letter requesting a change in the records is provided at the end of this chapter.

- A decision must be made about whether to comply with your request within a reasonable period of time. In most cases, there should be no difficulties with obtaining the information.

- If, for some reason, officials decide not to honor your request, you have a right to a hearing.

- Even if the school's decision stands, you can ask to include your own statement in the records.

As with medical information, although most professionals recognize your right to such information, in some cases you may encounter resistance. Try not to be intimidated if you encounter resistance. Simply explain that you understand that you are entitled to your child's educational records. If you are told that you wouldn't understand the report because it is highly technical, simply explain that you will ask questions about things you don't understand and that in the future you think that another professional may find it useful.

The records are useful for a number of reasons.

- First, if you change programs, service providers, or doctors or if you see a new specialist, it is helpful to have copies of those records available to give to new professionals. Although the new professional can, with your permission, obtain those copies directly from the previous program (or other professional), it may involve a wait of several days (even weeks). You can expedite the process by being able to provide those records yourself.

- Second, the records may help provide necessary documentation for insurance purposes or Medicaid.

- Third, if you find yourself involved in a due process hearing (see chapter 9), these records could be valuable as a way of documenting your position.

Summary of Developmental Milestones

As you see different professionals, you will probably be asked many questions about how well you think your child is doing. Many parents find they are asked the same questions over and over again. You may find it helpful to write it down when you notice that your child is doing something new. For example, a teacher, doctor or therapist may want to know when your child first held his head up, rolled over, sat up, said his first word, used a spoon, and so on. Don't worry if you don't think to write down everything you are asked about, or if you either didn't notice or can't remember everything. But if you notice, write it down. We recommend keeping your list in your file system. If and when someone asks you about a particular accomplishment, you won't have to guess. A list of developmental milestones that you may be asked about can be found in Table 2. This list is only intended to provide examples of the types of things you may be asked about. If you find you are consistently asked about other milestones, by all means add them to your list. We have found that it is easier to write them down than try to remember them later. It is easy to forget the age at which a specific milestone was achieved, even though it is a big accomplishment.

Communication Notebook

If your child receives home based services, you are probably in regular contact with the service providers who come to your home. As your child

---

Table 4-2
Common Milestones

AGE MY CHILD STARTED:
Smiling _____
Playing Peek-a-boo _____
Playing little games (e.g., pat-a-cake) _____
Making vowel sounds (ahh.., ohh...) _____
Making consonant sounds (bababa, dadada) _____
Using single words _____
Putting two words together _____
Making a sentence of three or more words _____
Turning to look at a sound _____
Holding up head _____
Rolling over _____
Sitting alone _____
Crawling _____
Walking (independently) _____
Walking up stairs _____
Jumping _____
Running _____
Sleeping through the night _____
Using a spoon (independently) _____
Using a fork (independently) _____
Drinking from a cup _____
Being Toilet Trained _____
Dressing himself/herself _____

---

grows and develops he or she may begin attending a center-based program — a school or therapeutic center where your child goes several days a week. Here too, you will be a valuable source of information for the teachers and therapists. Many parents find a communication notebook very helpful. You can note important events in your child's life which happen at home (e.g., has had a bad night, has been ill, is not eating well, has had a major change in routine, and so forth). You can also communicate information such as food likes and dislikes, new achievements that have been observed at home, relevant information from medical appointments and so forth.

Let the teacher know too, that you are interested in what kind of day your child has had at school. Some parents find it helpful to keep all of the notes from their child's teacher in one place. Later, they may help you review your child's progress, identify special needs and so forth.

It is especially important to keep your notes if you are experiencing any difficulties or inconsistencies in communication with professionals.

Crisis Plan

If you are a single parent or feel that you are the only person who is really aware of your child's routine and all of your child's needs, you may have concerns as to what might happen to your child if something were to happen to you. It may be helpful to write a letter outlining information about your child's medical care, medication, diagnoses, and professionals and programs involved with your child. Other critical information such as emergency numbers, insurance and Medicaid information might also be useful. Copies of this letter can be provided to relatives and placed in a conspicuous place in the house.

If there is any possibility that your child could experience a medical crisis, you should also place your own address and phone number, the telephone numbers of physicians in large letters near the telephone. In a crisis, it is easy to forget even your own address when you most need help. If other people are caring for your child at times, you may also want to place emergency contact numbers for yourself, your spouse, and other important persons near the phone. Finally, if your child is on an apnea monitor or may have a respiratory crisis, you may want to place a CPR poster near the crib or bed. **By calmly thinking through what to do in an emergency, you will be better prepared to act during a crisis.**

If your child is dependent on life support equipment, you may ask your hospital or home health nurse if they have forms to be sent to telephone and electrical companies in the event of a power outage. Your child's medical equipment typically has battery back-ups that will last for about four hours. Notices may be sent to the telephone and power companies stating that you have a child dependent upon electrical equipment, and your home will be given priority in restoration of telephone and power service. It is good too, to think through what **you** would need to do, in the event of an overnight power outage or telephone failure. This includes such things as transporting your baby to the hospital which will have a generator.

CONCLUSION

After reading the ideas described in this chapter, you will undoubtedly find some suggestions which are useful and others which cannot be applied to your particular situation. You may already have developed your own system. The details of how to set up your system is not as important as finding a way to access important information when the need for it arises. The key is to find something simple, easy to use, and readily accessible.

SAMPLE REQUEST FOR RECORDS
Dear (name of principal or program director),

My son(daughter), (child's name)   is currently enrolled in your program. At your earliest convenience, please provide written information concerning the records you have on   (child's name) . I would also like to know where you keep these records. Please provide me the name of a contact person and tell me how I can arrange to review (and make copies) of these records.

Thank you for your assistance with this matter.

Sincerely

SAMPLE REQUEST FOR CORRECTION OF RECORDS
Dear (name of program director or principal),

As I was reviewing   (child's name)   school records, I became concerned about the   (identify record)   dated   (give date) . I am concerned because I feel that the report is ... (give reason you feel report is inaccurate, violates your child's rights, etc).

I am requesting that the report be changed so that it no longer

Please notify me when this is changed and provide me with a changed copy that I can review.

Thank you,

CHAPTER 5

Educational Assessment

Paula J. Beckman, Joan Lieber, Janet Filer, & Diane Greig

Assessment is the process during which information is gathered about a child's development. Assessments take place for many different reasons. These reasons include making a diagnosis, making educational placements, designing educational programs, monitoring progress, and establishing the need for additional services. Assessments will occur repeatedly if you have a child who is developmentally delayed, disabled, or at risk for developmental delay.

For many parents, the process can seem mysterious and overwhelming. Since many important decisions about your child are based on the assessment results, it is worthwhile to know as much about this process as possible.

This chapter is intended to provide basic information about what assessments are and how they are conducted so as to remove some of the mystery. In this chapter we will describe: the areas of development which are typically assessed in young children, the steps in the assessment process, the professionals who are likely to assess each domain, the different types of assessment devices, the optimal conditions for assessment, your involvement in the assessment process, and how to make sense of the assessment report.

AREAS OF DEVELOPMENT
TYPICALLY ASSESSED IN YOUNG CHILDREN

Assessments cover many different areas of development which are often referred to as developmental domains. The domains which are generally assessed include cognitive, motor, language, social-emotional, and self-help development. In addition, if your child has a visual or hearing disability, there may be special assessments of these areas.

Cognitive development refers to your child's understanding of the world. This domain includes many different types of abilities. For example, you may hear your child's teacher or therapist use terms such as object permanence (remembering that something exists even if you can't see, hear, or touch it), means-end skills (using tools or people to solve problems), spatial relationships (recognizing an object's position in space), causality (understanding the cause of events), imitation (copying what others say or do), classification (sorting objects based on character-istics of the object like color, shape, or size), and matching (finding an object that is like another one). All of these are cognitive abilities that are likely to be assessed in your child.

Motor development. Motor development refers to your child's ability to move his body. Ideally, not only the presence or absence of motor skills should be assessed, but also the quality with which the movements are performed. Two types of motor development are usually differentiated by teachers and therapists. Gross motor refers to movement using the large muscles such as sitting, crawling, and walking. Fine motor refers to the ability to manipulate objects using eye-hand coordination. Fine motor skill is also involved in drawing and writing.

Language development refers to your child's ability to communicate. This includes spoken language as well as alternative forms such as sign language and communication boards. Two types of language develop-ment are frequently distinguished by professionals. Receptive language refers to the ability to understand others. Expressive language refers to the ability to use language with others.

Social-emotional development refers to your child's skills in developing and maintaining relationships with other people. Many different aspects of social-emotional development are considered by professionals de-pending on your child's age. Interactions with adults as well as with peers are included in social-emotional development.

Self-help development includes skills that allow your child to take care of his own daily needs. These abilities include self-feeding, toileting, groom-ing, and dressing. On some assessment instruments, social-emotional development and self-help skills are combined into an area called per-sonal-social abilities.

STEPS IN THE ASSESSMENT PROCESS

For children with disabilities, assessment is an on-going process that begins with the identification of a disability. Identification is only the beginning of what may sometimes seem like a never-ending process. Assessment continues for as long as your child is receiving services, and is used to monitor your child's progress and to identify new educational and therapeutic needs. A description of each of the major steps in the assessment process follows.

Screening

The first step is called *screening*. The purpose of screening is to determine in a quick, informal way whether your child is developing as expected. Children may be screened prior to kindergarten or during routine, well-baby visits. If you have concerns about your child's development, you may contact your local Child Find Office to request a screening.

A screening may include many different aspects of your child's health and development. It may be conducted by an educator, psychologist, physician, public health nurse, speech-language pathologist, physical therapist, occupational therapist, or trained paraprofessional. Physicians and nurses routinely screen your child's hearing, vision, and nutritional status. In addition, developmental screening determines how your child is functioning in the various developmental domains described earlier.

In developmental screening, children are observed and asked to do different tasks that are typical of children their age. The examiner may also ask you if your child is able to do certain things. For example, in a screening for motor development, the examiner may look to see if a baby can roll over or sit up. Preschool children may be asked to cut with scissors, hop on one foot, or throw a ball. When cognitive development is screened, babies might be asked to find something that is hidden or get an object that the examiner is holding. Preschool children may be asked to count blocks or identify colors. In screening language, a baby might be asked to imitate sounds or name simple, familiar objects. Preschool children pronounce words, identify pictures, or answer questions about how they would solve particular problems. In the personal-social area, your baby might be encouraged to play peek-a-boo or the examiner may ask you about your child's reaction to strangers. You might be asked whether your preschool child plays with others. In the self-help domain, you may be asked whether your child drinks from a cup, feeds himself, dresses himself, or is toilet-trained.

Screening is designed to be a brief look at your child's behavior, so the information that professionals can get from screening results is limited. Therefore, there are only two decisions that can be made as a result of screening. The first decision is that your child is developing normally and that further assessment is not needed. The second potential decision is that a problem may exist and further assessment is necessary.

If a child's disability is severe or if a clear disability has already been diagnosed, it is often unnecessary to do a screening. Parents of children with severe disabilities may already know that developmental problems exist. In these cases, screening is an unnecessary step in identification and intervention.

Diagnosis

The next step in the assessment process is diagnosis. Diagnostic testing is designed to determine if a child has a disability or a delay that requires intervention. In order to make this decision, the child's development and performance are compared to that of children of the same age who are developing normally. Diagnostic tests are more complex and take more time to administer than screening tests.

A medical diagnosis (such as Down syndrome or spina bifida) is usually made by a physician. A diagnosis of developmental delay may be made by a psychologist or a multidisciplinary team. This multidisciplinary team consists of a variety of professionals who have expertise in different areas of development. The team may include a special educator, a speech language pathologist, a physical therapist, an occupational therapist, a psychologist, a physician, an audiologist, an ophthalmologist, and a social worker. All these professionals are not members of every multidisciplinary team; membership depends on the needs of your child. However, as a parent, you should be included on your child's multidisciplinary team, because you have critical and unique knowledge about the development and performance of your child.

If your child is showing delays or has a disability, appropriate intervention and instructional strategies should be developed. Instructional objectives are determined during the next step of the assessment process.

Educational Assessment

The information that professionals get in order to make a diagnosis is not usually detailed enough to plan daily educational activities for children. The teachers and therapists who work with your child administer educational assessments in order to identify your child's strengths and weaknesses and plan your child's educational program.

It is especially important during this step of the assessment process that parents and professionals work together to determine instructional objectives. You can help professionals by describing what your child does at home, which is often very different than what professionals see during an assessment or at school. In addition, you can help professionals set priorities for your child's instructional program.

Using information from the educational assessment, the Individualized Education Program (IEP) or the Individual Family Service Plan (IFSP) will be written. These plans will be described in more detail in the next chapter.

Monitoring and Evaluating Instruction

The final step of the assessment process is one that continues the entire time that your child receives intervention. This step consists of regularly evaluating your child and her educational program to ensure that objectives are being met and that your child is developing and changing.

You are involved in monitoring in several ways. First, you will have the opportunity to meet periodically with professionals from your child's early intervention program to discuss progress on specific objectives and to decide when new objectives should be established. Second, you might be directly involved in intervention by working on your child's goals and objectives at home. As a result, you can provide information to professionals about your child's progress on objectives.

TYPES OF ASSESSMENTS

Many different types of assessments are used, depending on whether the purpose is screening, diagnosis, educational assessment, or monitoring. When children are assessed, their performance is sampled across the developmental domains described previously. Some instruments tap all of these areas while others are limited to just one particular area of development. Neisworth and Bagnato (1988) identify a number of different types of instruments and list some examples of each type. These types are described next.

Standardized or Norm-Referenced Instruments

Some assessment instruments are known as standardized or norm-referenced instruments. The term *standardized* is used because the materials and procedures are supposed to be the same for every child to whom they are given. They are called *norm-referenced* because they compare your child's performance to the performance of a group of other children at the same chronological age. Most tests of this type have not included children with disabilities as part of the comparison or norm group. When your child is evaluated using a norm-referenced instrument, she receives a score that represents her performance relative to others in the norm group. Some examples of commonly used norm-referenced instruments for young children are *The Battelle Developmental Inventory, The Bayley Scales of Infant Development,* and *The McCarthy Scales of Children's Abilities.* Standardized tests provide information about how similar your child is to a group of children without disabilities. However, these tests often provide little information to the teacher concerning specific educational goals. In addition, children with certain types of disabilities may be unable to respond to some items. For example, children with visual disabilities may not be able to respond to some items on a cognitive assessment which depend on vision. The inability to respond may have little or nothing to do with the cognitive ability that is being tested. The assessment report should acknowledge this limitation.

Criterion-Based or Criterion-Referenced Assessments. Another type of assessment device is known as a criterion-based or criterion-referenced test. Criterion-referenced tests are designed to evaluate children's strengths and weaknesses, rather than to compare their performance to the performance of other children. These instruments provide an in-depth understanding of children's abilities that teachers can use to plan instruction. Some examples of commonly used criterion-referenced instruments are the *BRIGANCE Diagnostic Inventory of Early Development,* the *Learning Accomplishment Profile* and the *Early Intervention Developmental Profile.*

Instruments with Adaptations. While norm and criterion-referenced instruments are used most commonly, other types of instruments may be used as well. For some children, particularly those with a sensory or a motor disability, it is difficult to accurately determine how they are progressing in a variety of developmental domains. Scales with adaptations for specific disabilities have been developed. For example, the *Oregon Project Curriculum* was designed for use with young children who have visual disabilities. In addition, other instruments provide the tester with directions on how to modify items. They may also allow children with particular disabilities to more easily demonstrate their abilities by using a different response. Both the *Battelle* and the *Early Intervention Developmental Profile* provide testers with information about these modifications.

Ecological Instruments. In addition to assessment instruments that focus specifically on the child's behavior, Neisworth & Bagnato (1988) identify other instruments which look more broadly at children in relationship to their environment. These instruments are called ecological assessment instruments. They enable parents and early interventionists to evaluate how different aspects of the environment influence development. Aspects of the environment include toys that your child plays with or opportunities for your child to interact with peers, caregivers and teachers. Two examples of ecological assessments are the *Home Observation for Measurement of the Environment* (HOME) and the *Early Childhood Environment Rating Scale*.

Systematic Observation. Finally, Neisworth & Bagnato (1988) identify some assessment procedures which rely on systematic observation of children in a variety of settings. When using systematic observation the examiner describes the behavior of interest, observes to see how often or for how long the behavior occurs, and describes the conditions under which the behavior occurs. These procedures allow both parents and early interventionists to collect information about children's behavior.

Interventionists use systematic observation when they want to increase or decrease certain behaviors or when they just want to describe the behavior that exists. For example, a teacher in the early intervention program may have noticed that Jason is hitting other children. In order to use systematic observation, the teacher would ask a series of questions including: how often does the hitting occur, does the hitting occur during specific times, what happens before Jason starts hitting, and what do the other children do in response to Jason's hitting.

Once the teacher has made a series of observations to answer those questions, she would be ready to intervene to decrease the hitting behavior. Interventionists use systematic observation to increase the frequency of such desirable behaviors as talking, playing with other children, and dressing independently.

OPTIMAL ASSESSMENT CONDITIONS

Since interventionists use assessments to make many important decisions about your child, assessments should be conducted under conditions which are best for your child. This is important to ensure that the information represents your child's true ability. Results may be affected by characteristics of your child, the examiner, the setting, and the procedures used.

Child Characteristics

Just as educational programming must be individualized — based upon the specific needs of your child, so must assessment. Except in the case of standardized tests, where uniform procedures and materials must be used, assessment methods should be matched to your child's needs. As we noted previously, children with sensory or physical disabilities may require adaptation of test materials and techniques. The examiner may use extra cues or prompts, as long as they will not interfere with the intent of the specific test item. For any child, but particularly for a child with a physical disability, the examiner should determine positioning and handling that will enhance performance. The age, temperament, and behavioral characteristics of your child determine the optimum amount of testing time. Direct testing periods should be limited for younger children and children who have difficulty in sustaining attention. Your child's "state" should also be considered carefully. State refers to the general level of alertness of your child and is influenced by such factors as medications, illness, time of day, and your child's schedule. Any of these factors can influence your child's performance. In addition, your child's interest in the specific materials used for testing will affect attention to the tasks and compliance with examiner requests.

Behavior of the Examiner

The examiner should respond to your child's mood and adjust the level of stimulation in the testing situation to your child's needs. You can provide the examiner with information about your child's use and understanding of communicative gestures and interactive style (Fewell, 1983). When feasible, assessments for educational programming should be conducted by an individual who knows your child, such as the teacher or therapist.

The Setting

The setting should be determined by the specific purpose for which the assessment is being given. If the purpose is to collect information on your child's social or communication skills, observational assessment in group settings is ideal. It is reasonable to question the accuracy of an assessment of social skills if the child is not observed in situations with other children. Conversely, if the purpose is to determine your child's performance on fine motor tasks, a setting free of distractions is optimal. Depending upon your child, your presence during the assessment may or may not enhance your child's performance (Bailey & Wolery, 1984).

Assessment Procedures

To get a good representation of your child's abilities, an assessment which is conducted for educational programming should not be limited to any single setting, tester, or time period, because your child will often behave differently in different places, with different people and at different times during the day. The assessment process should include a team of professionals from a variety of disciplines and at least one parent or guardian. The combined assessments of a variety of professionals and the parent(s) provide the most comprehensive and representative picture of your child's abilities.

PARENT INVOLVEMENT IN THE ASSESSMENT

As a parent, you can play an important and active role in the assessment process. If possible, make an effort to observe the assessment yourself.

This will be relatively easy if your child is in a home program or if you take your child to a clinic for an evaluation. If your child is in a preschool placement, observing may be somewhat more difficult since the assessment may take place during the school day. However, you may be able to make arrangements with the teacher or therapist to watch the assessment.

As you are observing the assessment, it may help to keep a pad of paper handy on which you can jot questions. However, if you must hold your child, this may not be a realistic possibility. While the assessment is taking place, mentally ask yourself some questions. For example, is your child in a comfortable position that will permit his best responses? Would he have been better able to complete the task or activity at home or with different objects, toys or materials? Are there other circumstances under which your child is likely to perform the task more effectively? Is your child distracted so much by something in the room that it is interfering with his performance? If the answer to any of these questions is yes, be sure to tell the examiner. This will help the examiner interpret your child's performance more accurately.

Be sure to tell the examiner about anything else that might influence your child's performance. For example, if your child is cutting teeth, she may show as much interest in chewing or mouthing test materials as in performing the task. This will also help the examiner to interpret the findings. If you feel that your child is not performing at her best, you may want to have the assessment rescheduled for another time. In other instances, you may just want to inform the teacher or examiner to make certain that this information is included in the interpretation of the results.

Finally, when you discuss the assessment with the professionals who gave it, there are a number of questions which you may want to consider asking.

1. What was the name of the assessment my child was given? Once you know the name of the assessment, you can look it up in the descriptions provided in Table 1. These descriptions provide basic information regarding the most commonly used assessment devices in early intervention and in some related fields.

2. What is the purpose of the assessment? As indicated earlier, assessments are given for many different reasons Assessments conducted in order to determine placement decisions can have an important influence on your child's future. In such cases, it may be important to reschedule the assessment if your child is not feeling well or is having an especially bad day so that the examiner can get the best possible picture of your child's skills.

3. What areas of development does the assessment measure? Some assessment instruments focus specifically on one area of development while others cover many different developmental domains. Professionals may administer a battery of tests in order to make certain that all areas of your child's development are evaluated. Decisions about your child's abilities should be made considering the whole child. While assessments which focus on only one area of development are often very good, it is important to make sure that all of your child's needs are assessed. If you think your child has needs which have not been addressed, it is important to bring that to the attention of the professional team and to ask for an assessment of that area.

4. Was this particular assessment device appropriate given my child's disability? First, is the assessment device intended for use with children who have your child's disability? Second, were modifications made to accommodate your child's disability?

5. What positive changes or strengths did you see? Sometimes in the process of assessment, it is easy to focus more on what the child didn't do than what she did do. By asking this question you can make sure that you get a balanced perspective about your child and can force everyone to focus on positive aspects of your child's performance instead of only on the things she is not doing. Under the most recent Part H regulations, assessment is intended to include an assessment of the child's strengths as well as needs. You can make sure this happens by asking the question directly.

MAKING SENSE OF THE ASSESSMENT REPORT

The purpose of an assessment report is to summarize the results of test information. This information is used to make a diagnosis or to make recommendations about an appropriate intervention program. Although

Table 5-1
Early Childhood Assessment

Name of Instrument	Purpose	Type of Instrument	Domains	Age Range	Adaptations for Disabilities
Battelle Developmental Inventory (BDI) Newborg, Stock, Wnek, Guidubald & Svenick, 1984. Texas: DLM Teaching Resources	assessment and educational programming	criterion-referenced and norm-referenced	personal-social, motor (gross and fine), communication (receptive and expressive), adaptive (self-help) and cognitive	birth to 8 years	yes — allows response most appropriate for child's disability
Brigance Inventory of Early Development Brigance, 1979. Curriculum Associates, Inc.	educational programming	crtierion-referenced	preambulatory motor skills and behaviors, gross motor, fine motor, self-help, speech and language, general knowledge, social emotional, readiness, basic reading, manuscript, and basic math	birth to seven years	yes
Brigance Inventory of Basic Skills Brigance, 1979. Curriculum Associate, Inc.	educational programming	criterion-referenced	readiness reading, language, arts, and math	K-6th grade	yes
Receptive-Expressive Emergent Language Scale (REEL) Bzock & League, 1970. Baltimore, MD: University Park Press	screening	norm-referenced	receptive and expressive language, prelinguistic skills	birth to 36 months	no

Name of Instrument	Purpose	Type of Instrument	Domains	Age Range	Adaptations for Disabilities
Carolina Curriculum for Infants and Toddlers with Special Needs Johnson-Martin, Jens, Attermeier, & Hacker, 1991. Baltimore, MD: Paul H. Brookes	educational programming and curriculum	curriculum-referenced	cognition, communication, social adaptation, fine motor and gross motor	birth to 2	yes
Carolina Curriculum for Preschoolers with Special Needs Johnson-Martin, Jens, Attermeier, & Hacker, 1991. Baltimore, MD: Paul H. Brookes	educational programming and curriculum	curriculum-referenced	cognition, communication, social adaptation, fine motor and gross motor	2 to 5 years	yes
Denver Developmental Screening Test II Frankenburg & Dodds, 1990. Colorado: Denver Developmental Materials	screening	norm-referenced	personal-social, fine motor, gross motor, adaptive, and language	2 weeks to 6.4 years	no
Dial-R (Developmental Indicators for The Assessment of Learning Revised) Mardell-Czudnowski & Goldenberg, 1983.	screening	norm-referenced	motor, language, conceptual	2-6 years	no
Early Intervention Developmental Profile (EIDP) Schafer & Moersch, 1981. University of Michigan Press	educational programming	curriculum-referenced	perceptual.fine motor, cognition, language, social/emotional, self-care, gross motor	birth to 36 months and 35 to 60 months	yes — adapted for children with visual, hearing, and neuro-motor disabilities
Education of Multihandicapped Infants (EMI) Elder & Swift, 1975. Virginia: University of Virginia, Department of Pediatrics	educational programming	criterion-referenced	gross motor, fine motor, social, cognition, and language	birth to 24 months	

Table 5-1 (cont.)

Name of Instrument	Purpose	Type of Instrument	Domains	Age Range	Adaptations for Disabilities
Early Learning Accomplishment profile (ELAP) Glover, Preminger, & Sanford, 1978. North Carolina: Kaplan School Supply	educational programming	curriculum-referenced	gross motor, fine motor, cognition, language, self-help, social-emotional	birth to 36 months	no
Milani-Comparetti Motor Development Screening Revised, Trembath, 1977. Nebraska: Meyer Children's Rehabilitation Institute	screening	criterion-referenced	motor development	birth to 2 years	no
Gesell Developmental Language Scales Revised, Knoblock, Stevens, & Malone, 1987. Texas: Developmental Evaluation Materials	educational programming	norm-referenced	language development	1 to 7 years	
Vineland Adaptive Behavior Scales, Sparrow, Bella, & Cicchetti, 1984. Minnesota: American Guidance Service	evaluation and diagnosis; educational programming	norm-referenced	communication, daily living skills, socialization, and motor skills	birth to 18 years 11 months or a low functioning adult	has been used with disabled individuals 6 to 40 years with mental retardation, visual impairment, and learning impairment

Name of Instrument	Purpose	Type of Instrument	Domains	Age Range	Adaptations for Disabilities
Bayley Scales of Infant Development, Bayley, 1969. New York: Psychological Corporation	assessment of the developmental progress of infants	norm-referenced	motor scale, mental scale, social and objective orientation scale	birth to 30 months	no
Early Language Milestone Scale, Coplan, 1983. Oklahoma: Modern Education Corporation	screening	norm-referenced	language - auditory expressive, auditory receptive, and visual	birth to 36 months	no, but has been validated with high risk and developmentally delayed children
Transdisciplinary Play-Based Assessment, Linder, 1990. Maryland: Paul H. Brooks.	educational programming	criterion-referenced	cognitive, social-emotional, communication and language, and sensorimotor development	6 months to 6 years	yes, it can be individualized for children with disabilities
Preschool Language Scale-3 (PLS-3), Zimmerman, Steiner, & Pond, 1992. Psychological Corporation, Harcourt Brace Jovanovick, Inc.	assessment	norm-referenced	receptive and expressive language	birth to 6 years 11 months	yes, but if you alter the administration directions, it can only be used as a criterion-referenced measure
Brazelton Neonatal Assessment Scale, Brazelton, 1984. Pennsylvania: J.B. Lippincott	assess behavioral and neurological status of newborn; educational programming with parents.	screening	assesses newborn's reflexes and interactive behaviors	3 days to 6 weeks	

there is a typical format for presentation of assessment information, there may be some variation in any individual report (Sattler, 1988).

Identifying Information

This section of the assessment report provides information such as the name, address, birth date of the child, parents' names, the name of the examiner, the setting in which the tests were administered, and the names of the tests.

Reason for the Referral

The section includes the source of the referral. For example, the child might be referred by the parents, by the Child Find Office, or by a pediatrician. In addition, this section includes a summary of questions and concerns about development that indicate the need for assessment.

Background Information

This section relies heavily on information given by caregivers in interviews. It includes details about the child such as the birth history, medical background, and achievement of major developmental milestones. For example, discussion of when the child began walking, or using language to communicate would appear here. This section also includes any relevant family information.

Behavioral Observations

This section describes how the child behaved during the testing situation itself. If a statement is made about the child's behavior, there should also be examples given to support the statement. For example, if the child is described as uncooperative in the testing situation, there should also be specific examples given to support the statement such as, "Mary was generally uncooperative during test administration. She was unable to settle at the table for structured testing. She often ran away to get toys on the other side of the room. In addition, when test materials were presented, she threw them on the floor." In this section, the evaluator has the opportunity to generally describe the child and may include information about the child's activity level, reactions to testing, and responses to success or failure.

Assessment Results

In this section of the assessment report, the evaluator discusses results of the tests that were administered. It may be organized based on the results of each test, or the results from a variety of tests may be combined based on performance in each developmental domain. For example, all the motor information may be combined together even if it comes from a variety of tests and observations. The examiner may describe your child's performance in terms of an exact score or in terms of a range of scores.

Even when test scores are reported, it is important that the evaluator does more than report scores on a particular test. There should be descriptions of the child's strengths and weaknesses, and indications that result from testing are confirmed by other information. For example, if a language assessment shows that "Juanita uses gestures to request a toy," this should be confirmed with information from parents as well.

Summary and Recommendations

The final section of the assessment report provides a summary of all the information presented. In this section of the report, the evaluator also makes recommendations as to possible placement in an intervention program and possible goals of the program. It is important to remember that the evaluator is presenting only one point of view. At the multidisciplinary team meeting, all participants come together to present their findings, and there may be differences of opinion about what type of intervention program is needed.

CONCLUSION

As we noted earlier, the process of obtaining an assessment may often seem rather difficult and complicated. For example, professionals may insist on testing your child in a certain way or may not always give your child credit for some things that you know he can do. The purpose of this chapter has been to provide you with basic information about assessment in order to demystify the process for you. Hopefully, we have helped you understand some of the procedures that professionals use. It should be noted that the assessment procedures described above are ideal; you may find differences in the way your child is assessed and in the procedures used by your school or early intervention program. However, knowledge of the most appropriate procedures and the reasons they are used should help you to determine if a realistic evaluation of your child's skills has been obtained.

REFERENCES

Bagnato, S.J., Neisworth, J.T., & Munson, S. M. (1989). *Linking developmental assessment and early intervention: Curriculum-based prescription.* Rockville, MD: Aspen.

Bailey, D.B., & Wolery, M. (1984). *Teaching infants and preschoolers with handicaps.* Columbus, OH: Merrill.

Bailey, D.B., & Wolery, M. (1989). *Assessing infants and preschoolers with handicaps.* Columbus, OH: Merrill.

Fewell, R.R. (1983). Assessing handicapped infants. In S.G. Garwood & R.R. Fewell (Eds.) *Educating handicapped infants: Issues in development and intervention* (pp. 257-297).

Neisworth, J.T., & Bagnato, S.J. (1988). Assessment in early childhood special education: A typology of dependent measures. In S.L. Odom & M.B. Karnes (Eds.). *Early intervention for infants and children with handicaps* (pp. 23- 49). Baltimore: Paul H. Brookes.

Sattler, J. M. (1988). *Assessment of children* (3rd ed.). San Diego: Joel M. Sattler, Publisher.

CHAPTER 6

Gathering Information about Your Family

Paula J. Beckman, Sandra Newcomb, Vera Stroup and Cordelia Robinson

At some point, particularly if your child is less than three years of age, the service providers you encounter are likely to request information from you about your family. In most cases, this information is collected in response to the federal requirement that family concerns, priorities and resources should be incorporated in the Individual Family Service Plan. Providing this information is voluntary on your part and is to be included with your consent. This chapter is intended to describe why information about families is important, what you should communicate, the kind of information which may be requested, ways family information is collected, and the questions you should ask.

Why Gather Information About Families?

There are many important reasons early intervention personnel may request information about your family. The most important reason is that professionals have begun to recognize that your child is part of a larger system, your family. (Dunst, Trivette and Deal, 1988; Robinson, Rosenberg, & Beckman, 1988; Turnbull, Summers, & Brotherson, 1986). Your family, in turn, is part of a larger community. Anything that interventionists recommend for your child is going to affect more than just your child, it will affect everyone else in your family as well. There are many examples of this impact. If you have to take your child to many different appointments (e.g., for doctors, therapists, etc.) you may have to rearrange your schedule, have difficulty maintaining a regular work schedule, or have less time to spend with other family members. Concern about services for your child may influence a decisions to accept employment that would require your family to relocate. If your child has a behavior problem, you may find yourself avoiding social situations that would test the limits of your child's ability to cope.

Similarly, as part of a larger community, circumstances that affect you and other family members may also have an influence on your child. If you are extremely tired or anxious, you may find that your child senses this. If you work outside your home, you may be less available to participate in your child's school activities or may have less time to work on activities with your child. Other children in the family have needs that compete for time and resources with those of your child with a disability.

It is important for early intervention personnel to be aware of these issues. Relatively small changes can often be implemented by your child's service providers which make your life much easier. For, example, if you work during the day, your teacher may be able to arrange home visits in the evening. You may find there are additional services available that can help in the very area in which you are having difficulties.

Increased recognition of the mutual effect that children with disabilities and their families have on one another has resulted in many of the service requirements that have been described in other chapters. One requirement for states that are implementing programs for infants and toddlers under Part H is that programs must identify family concerns, priorities and resources when they are planning programs for children from birth through age two years. Your own concerns, priorities, and resources may be quite similar to those of other families. On the other hand, your particular circumstances may result in unique concerns and needs. Your family may also bring unique strengths and resources to the situation. As a result, intervention programs are developing ways to learn about your family's circumstances so that this knowledge can be incorporated into the plans for your child and family.

In general, the information which is collected should be family directed, voluntary on the part of the family, conducted by persons trained to use appropriate methods and procedures, and include a personal interview. Make sure that you get *your* opinions across to the team of individuals who will be providing services to your child and family.

What Should You to Communicate?

The process of formally identifying family concerns, priorities, and resources is an important opportunity to have input into the services that are provided for your child and family. There are many things you may wish to communicate. Early interventionists can plan services that meet your needs better if you give them an idea about what life with your child is like and what your concerns are about your child. In addition, some concerns are likely to be more important to you than others. Let service providers know what your priorities are. For example, one of your top priorities may be that you want your child to attend kindergarten with children who do not have disabilities. By making the early intervention- ist aware that this is your priority, the interventionist can focus on your child's social skills and other activities that may increase the likelihood of kindergarten attendance later. The service coordinator can help iden- tify any special assistance that your child may need in order to participate in kindergarten. Special activities can be planned which will promote success in kindergarten (for example, special sessions with nondisabled peers to answer their questions about your child's disability).

It is also important to make sure that interventionists have a clear idea of your family's beliefs and values. This is especially important if your culture and background are different from those of the professionals serving you. Given the range of religions, races, and ethnic traditions represented in the United States, you cannot always assume that profes- sionals will be familiar with your culture, beliefs, and values. Sharing these values will give professionals a better understanding of your decisions and help them provide services that are consistent with your priorities and values.

Types of Information Collected

During the family interview, several types of information are typically requested. The most common are questions about your child's or family's concerns, priorities, and/or needs as well as resources and supports. In some cases interventionists may also ask about any stresses or pressures that your family is experiencing and about your interactions with your child.

Family Concerns, Priorities, and Needs. Asking about family concerns, priorities and/or needs involves finding out what is needed to help your child develop to his or her potential. The purpose of sharing this informa- tion is to help determine what early intervention services your family will receive. There are several types of family concerns.

- Family concerns may be related only to your child and his or her disability such as concern about specific services (e.g., speech therapy) or the need for the child to learn specific skills (e.g., how to feed herself).

- Family concerns may also relate to the day-to-day functioning of your family because there is a child who has a disability. These needs would include such things as day care for a child with special needs or special seating so the child can travel outside of the home.

- Sometimes family concerns are more general and are not related to the fact that the child has a disability. For example, you may need housing or transportation to get groceries.

All of these are family concerns and may be discussed with a professional at the family interview or at any time you think it is appropriate. Although the agencies with whom you are working are not necessarily responsible for meeting all of these needs (particularly the more general needs), you may find it helpful to discuss them with your service coordinator or other members of the team. These individuals may be able to refer you to a service that could provide assistance to your family. Just knowing that you are facing other concerns may give service providers a better appreciation of your situation and its effect on other aspects of your life.

While you are discussing your concerns and/or needs, be sure to identify which needs are the *most important* to you at the time. Knowing your priorities will give professionals an idea of where they can begin their work. What do you want for your child now? Where do we start? There are several published instruments which service providers may use to help them identify your priorities, concerns and needs. Some of these measures are described in Table 6-1 to give you an idea of what these instruments are like.

Family Strengths, Resources and Supports. The purpose of sharing information about your family's strengths, resources, and/or supports is to build on the existing strengths that families have and to determine where new or additional services may be most useful. Families often have many resources and supports (Robinson, et al., 1988). Some resources are tangible, such as housing, food, and clothing. The support you receive from family members, friends, neighbors and professionals is also a

Table 6-1
Family Concerns, Priorities and Needs

Instrument	Description
Family Needs Survey (Bailey and Simeonsson, 1988)	This measure assesses the parents' need for information, social support, help explaining to others, financial assistance, child care assistance, professional support, and community services. Parents indicate whether they would like to talk about this with someone and how much assistance they may need within a given area on a one to three scale.
Caregiving Questionnaire (Beckman, 1980)	Parents indicate the extent to which their child has special needs in the area of feeding, handling and medical care.
Family Needs Scale (Dunst, Cooper, Weeldreyer, Snyder and Chase, 1988)	This scale measures the family's need for different types of resources and support. Parents do this by rating their needs in areas such as child care, financial, and food and shelter. Parents rate items on a 5-point scale ranging from almost never need (1) to almost always need (5).

resource and often a great source of strength. Some of this support may be emotional (e.g., people you can talk to about your child and family). Sometimes support can be more concrete (e.g., people who will babysit for your child, or give you rides to appointments).

- You may be asked to describe individuals who are supportive in your life or you may be given a list of possible sources of support and asked to describe how helpful each one is.

- Many people find it helpful to think about the strategies they use that help them cope. Since different people have different coping styles, it is important to focus on what is actually helpful to you. For example, some people find it helpful to talk to friends. Others find reading helpful. Others may seek information from different professionals before making decisions.

- What helps *you* cope with the concerns that arise in your life? Do you have a good sense of humor? Do you take pride in the small accomplishments of your child? Do you take comfort in your religion? Does everyone in your family pitch in and help when there is a problem? Are you highly organized? These qualities are all resources. They are very valuable characteristics that are part of the way that you and your family will work with professionals.

Family Stress. Sometimes service providers may ask about stresses or pressures that are placed on you and your family. Questions about family stress are usually asked in order to better understand the issues and events that affect your family and to better identify your needs or concerns. There are a number of measures designed to evaluate family stress. However, some of the questions may seem quite personal and seem to have little relevance to your child's program. As a result, many programs do not collect such information. If yours does, and you feel that this information is relevant, by all means answer the questions. However, you are not obliged to answer any of these questions. If you are uncomfortable or don't see how the questions relate to your child's program, feel free to tell the service provider that you are uncomfortable and do not wish to complete the form or to answer individual questions.

Parent-Child Interaction. Information on parent-child interaction is collected for a variety of reasons. Professionals may be interested in knowing how your child plays, how your child communicates, and the ways that you use to teach your child various tasks. Programs sometimes use information about the ways parents and children interact to get ideas about activities that a child enjoys, ways that a child learns, and methods that a parent has found effective in working with their own child. For example, you may know that your child prefers a special toy and may work harder to get it.

Table 6-2
Family Strengths, Resources and Supports

Instrument	Description
Carolina Parent Support Scale (Bristol, 1986)	Families rate the helpfulness of certain types of support that parents receive from professionals, relatives, or other parents. Sources of support are rated on a scale from 0 (not helpful) to 4 (extremely helpful).
Family Functioning Style Scale (Deal, Trivette and Dunst, 1988)	This scale measures: 1) different family qualities (e.g., coping strategies) and 2) how different combinations of strengths define the family's functioning style. Parents rate the extent to which different statements are like their family and identify what they consider to be their family strengths.
Family Support Scale (Dunst, Jenkins and Trivette, 1988)	Parents rate the helpfulness of different sources of support (e.g.spouse, friends, other parents) when raising a child with a disability on a (1) (not at all helpful) to (5) (extremely helpful) scale.
Family Resource Scale (FRS) (Dunst and Leet,1987)	Families rate the adequacy of basic resources (such as food, housing, child care, special equipment) on a 5-point scale ranging from not at all adequate (1) to almost always adequate (5).
Support Functions Scale (Dunst and Trivette, 1988)	This scale lists the various types of support parents may need in order to cope with the additional stressors of having a child with a disability. Parents rate how often they need help with each item on a 5-point scale ranging from never (1) to quite often (5).

continued on next page

Table 6-2 (cont.)

Instrument	Description
Profile of Family Needs and Supports (Dunst, Trivette and Deal, 1988)	This measure provides a way of recording particular resources and support services for families' needs, projects and aspirations. Parents identify needs and projects as well as sources of support of meeting their needs.
Family Strengths Profile (Dunst, Trivette and Deal, 1988)	This checklist examines the particular characteristics that best describe the family, noting the family's particular strengths and resources that the behavior reflects.
Coping Health Inventory for Parents (McCubbin, McCubbin, Nevin and Cauble, 1979)	This scale measures parents' perceptions of how they respond to the management of their life when they have a child who is seriously ill. This scale focuses primarily the parents' coping behaviors. Parents indicate the extent to which each of the coping strategies identified is helpful.
Personal Network Matrix (Trivette and Dunst, 1988)	This scale determines the types of individuals, agencies and groups the family has contact with and how these are used to support the family's needs, aspirations or projects.
Inventory of Social Support (Trivette and Dunst, 1988)	On this measure the responses indicate the frequency of contact with individuals in the personal support network (e.g., spouse, friends) and who they go to for specified types of help and assistance (e.g., who helps with house-hold chores, who provides encouragement).

Table 6-3
Family Stress Measures

Instrument	Description
Parenting Stress Index (Abidin, 1983)	Parents rate the magnitude of stress associated with parenting on a strongly agree (1) to strongly disagree (5) scale.
Questionnaire on Resources and Stress (Holroyd, 1986)	Parents indicate on a true/false scale the way in which the child with a disability or a chronic illness affects the family.
Family Inventory of Life Events and Changes (McCubbin and Patterson, 1987)	This scale measures the accumulations of life events over the last 12 months. Mothers and fathers complete separate forms for their families.
Impact-on-Family Scale (Stein and Reissman, 1990)	This instrument measures the impact of a chronically ill child on the family. The questions are related to the parent-child system and the child's illness.

Professionals may also be able to offer information, suggestions and feedback to you regarding new approaches that may work with your child, such as ideas about different ways to position your child that may make routine tasks such as diapering or feeding easier.

Information about parent-child interaction may be evaluated through a questionnaire or through direct observation. If you are unsure why such information is being collected, *ask*! If you are uncomfortable for any reason, you are free to decline.

Ways Family Information Is Collected.

Although most professionals now recognize the importance of incorporating information about family concerns, priorities and resources, there are a variety of ways that such information may be gathered.

Interviews. One way professionals obtain information about your family is through the use of informal interviews. Many parents feel more comfortable simply talking to professionals about their concerns than they do completing paper and pencil measures. During an interview, the interventionist is likely to ask general questions about your concerns, priorities and resources. This process allows you to include whatever information that you decide is appropriate. For example, the interviewer may simply ask you to tell them about your child. Such interviews have the advantage of allowing both participants to clarify issues and allowing you to expand in areas which are of most concern to you.

Interviews can be either structured or unstructured. In structured interviews, the service provider is likely to have a predefined set of questions that he or she brings to the visit. If this is the case, and the interviewer does not bring up a topic which is of concern to you, *do not hesitate to raise the issue yourself.*

Other interviews may be less structured and seem more like a conversation. If this is the case and you are unclear as to how the information will be used, speak up! By knowing the purpose, you can give the service provider more relevant information. During an interview, the information you provide about your concerns, priorities and resources will be identified as you talk. If you are unclear as to the conclusions that are being drawn, ask the professional to summarize or review his or her perceptions. This will give you the opportunity to clarify misconceptions and provide additional, relevant information if it is needed.

Observations. Some service providers may ask to observe you during interactions with your child. Observations are done in several ways. A professional may ask to come to your home and watch you and your child during every day activities. Or they may set up a task, situation or activity and ask you to do something specific. For example, they may show you a task and ask you to teach it to your child.

There are many reasons that such a request may be made. One reason is that parent-child interactions are believed to be one of the major ways in which young children learn. In some cases, children with disabilities do not use the same cues or signals that other children use. However, they may use *other* cues that provide the caregiver with important information. By observing the way that parents and children interact, professionals can obtain important information about the way that a particular child communicates his or her needs. Parents and teachers can learn from each other about the cues that work and those that do not.

The teacher or therapist may also be able to give information about the way in which a disability may influence interactions. For example, you may not understand why your child who has a visual impairment seems to see you sometimes and not others. However, once you understand that your child's vision is limited when he or she tries to look to the left or down, the reasons for his inconsistent responses may be clearer. You can then alter your behavior by making sure you are within his visual range when you play with him or ask him to look at a picture or an object.

Questionnaires. Another way that may be used to gather information about your family is through the use of paper and pencil measures. Questionnaires may be used as a supplement or as an integral part of the interview. These tools typically ask you to respond to a predetermined set of questions. Your responses may be limited to true-false responses; you may be asked to rate the extent to which specific items represent your family on a scale of three or more, or you may simply be asked to check when particular items apply to your family. Questionnaires allow service providers to do several things. In some cases, questionnaires are used to collect information about concerns, needs, priorities, stress, resources, strengths and/or supports. Sometimes questionnaires are used to evaluate the success of the intervention program. Other times they are used to compare your responses to those of a larger group. Your responses will then form the basis for further discussion and planning of intervention services.

Questions to Ask Professionals

Remember that the information a program collects about your family should be obtained at your discretion and with your consent. You may share what you want. You do *not* have to provide information that you do not want to share or are uncomfortable sharing.

As you talk with service providers, ask yourself how the information relates to your child's development. The information should have a purpose related to early intervention with your child. For example, if your child has asthma, you may want to describe things such as whether or not you have a family pet or whether your house is carpeted. This information is related to your child and her disability. The same information may not be as relevant if your child has Down syndrome. The questions asked and the information you share should be related to your child, her disability, or conditions in your family that affect how you deal with your child.

If you feel at any time that the professional is asking for information that you do not want to share (for example, detailed information about your marriage), you have the right not to answer. You can say, "I don't feel comfortable discussing that right now," or "I'm not sure how that question is related to my child's development (or progress or intervention, etc.)."

Even when you are very comfortable sharing information about your child and family, be sure you know how the information is recorded and used. You should feel free to ask, "What is the purpose of this question?" "How will you use the information?" Also find out if the service provider is taking notes. If so, ask whether a report is being written and find out who will see it. If you don't want the information shared, you should make that clear. If a report is written, request copies for your records.

Conclusion

Early intervention is a partnership of parents and professionals. To have an effective partnership, there must be an open exchange of information. The process of defining family concerns, priorities, and resources and designing an effective intervention for your child and family occurs over time as you work together with early intervention service providers. The process of early intervention is a dialogue in which each partner is free to share information. Feel free to share or not share whatever information you choose about your child and family. Ask service providers to share what they observe about your child and what they know about other children in similar situations or with similar disabilities. The process of gathering information about your family should be positive and nonintrusive. It is intended to help interventionists tailor services to meet the needs of your child and family in the most effective way possible.

REFERENCES

Abbott, D. and Meredith, W. (1986). Strengths of parents with retarded children. *Family Relations, 35, 371-375.*

Abidin, R.R. (1986). Parenting stress index (2nd ed.). Charlottesville, VA: Pediatric Psychology Press.

Bailey, D. and Wolery, M. (1989). *Assessing infants and preschoolers with handicaps.* Columbus, Ohio: Merrill Publishing Company.

Bailey, D. and Simeonsson, R. (1988). *Family assessment in early intervention.* Columbus, Ohio: Merrill Publishing Company.

Bristol, M. (1987). Carolina Parent Support Scale. Methodological caveats in the assessment of single-parent families of handicapped children. *Journal for the Divison of Early Childhood, 11, 135-142.*

Deal, A. Dunst, C., Trivette, C.,(1988). Family Functioning Style Scale. In C. Dunst, C. Trivette & A. Deal (Eds.), *Enabling and Empowering Families: Principles and guidelines for practice.* Cambridge, MA: Brookline Books.

Dunst, C., Cooper, C., Weeldreyer, J., Snyder, K., and Chase, J. (1988). Family Needs Scale. In C. Dunst, C. Trivette & A. Deal (Eds.), *Enabling and Empowering Families: Principles and guidelines for practice.* Cambridge, MA: Brookline Books.

Dunst, C., Jenkins, V., Trivette, C. (1988). Inventory of Social Support. In C. Dunst, C. Trivette & A. Deal (Eds.), *Enabling and Empowering Families: Principles and guidelines for practice.* Cambridge, MA: Brookline Books.

Dunst, C. and Leet, H.D. (1987). Family Resource Scale. In C. Dunst, C. Trivette & A. Deal (Eds.), *Enabling and Empowering Families: Principles and guidelines for practice.* Cambridge, MA: Brookline Books.

Dunst, C. and Trivette, C. (1988). Inventory of Social Support. In C. Dunst, C. Trivette & A. Deal (Eds.), *Enabling and Empowering Families: Principles and guidelines for practice.* Cambridge, MA: Brookline Books.

Dunst, C. and Trivette, C. (1988). Personal Network Matrix. In C. Dunst, C. Trivette & A. Deal (Eds.), *Enabling and Empowering Families: Principles and guidelines for practice.* Cambridge, MA: Brookline Books.

Dunst, C. and Trivette, C. (1988). Support Function Scale. In C. Dunst, C. Trivette & A. Deal (Eds.), *Enabling and Empowering Families: Principles and guidelines for practice.* Cambridge, MA: Brookline Books.

Dunst, C., Trivette, C., and Deal, A. (1988). Profile of Family Needs and Supports. In C. Dunst, C. Trivette & A. Deal (Eds.), *Enabling and Empowering Families: Principles and guidelines for practice.* Cambridge, MA: Brookline Books.

Dunst, C., Trivette, C., and Deal, A. (1988). *Enabling and Empowering Families: Principles and guidelines for practice.* Cambridge, MA: Brookline Books.

Holroyd, J. (1986). Questionnaire on resources and stress for families with chronically ill or handicapped member: Manual. Brandon, VT: Clinical Psychology Publishing.

Lewis, J., Beavers, W., Gossett, J. and Austin-Phillips, V. (1976). Family system rating scales. In J. Lewis et al. *No single thread: Psychological health in family systems.* New York: Brunner/Mazel.

McCubbin, McCubbin, Nevin and Cauble (1979). Coping Health Inventory for Parents. In H.I. McCubbin & A.I. Thompson (Eds.), *Family assessment inventories for research and practice.* Madison: University of Wisconsin.

McCubbin, H., and Patterson, J.M. (1987). Family Inventory of Life Events and Changes. In H.M. McCubbin and A.I. Thompson (Eds.) *Family assessment inventories for research and practice_*(pp.79-98). Madison: University of Wisconsin-Madison.

Olson, D., Portner, J., and Bell, R. (1982). Family adaptation and cohesion evaluation scales. Unpublished rating scales. School of Family and Social Sciences, University of Minnesota, St. Paul.

Pascoe, Loda, Jeffries and Earp (1981). The association between mothers' social support and provision of stimulation to their children. *Developmental and Behavioral Pediatrics, 2, 15-19.*

Robinson, C.C. , Rosenberg, S.A., and Beckman, P.J. (1988). Parent involvement in early childhood special education. In J. B. Jordan, J. J. Gallagher, P.L. Hutinger, and M. B. Karnes (Eds.) *Early childhood special education: Birth to three.*

Reston, VA: Council for Exceptional Children

Stein, R.E., and Reissman, C.K. (1980). The development of an impact-on-family scale: Preliminary findings. *Medical Care, 18, 465-472.*

Turnbull, A.P., Summers, J. A., & Brotherson, M. J. (1986). Family life cycle. In A.P. Turnbull & H. R. Turnbull (Eds.) *Families, professionals, and exceptionality: A special partnership.* Columbus, OH: Merrill Publishing.

CHAPTER 7

The IEP/IFSP Meeting

Paula J. Beckman, Gayle Boyes and Abigail Herres

An important part of recent legislation on behalf of young children who have disabilities is the meeting to discuss the Individual Education Plan (IEP) or Individual Family Service Plan (IFSP). In general, IEPs are required for children three years of age or more whereas IFSPs are required for children from birth through age two. In some cases, local education agencies may elect to use an IFSP for children from three to five. These plans form the basis of your child's intervention program. They are required to ensure that the services provided for each child and family are tailored individually for them. They will be developed and reviewed in annual or semi-annual meetings that you have with the service providers who are involved with your child.

Differences Between the IEP and the IFSP

The Individual Education Plan (IEP). The IEP is an educational plan required for all children with disabilities who are three years old or more (unless the local school system decides to use an IFSP). Services for children in this age range are the responsibility of the public schools; thus the IEP will be designed jointly by you and the professionals from your child's school or intervention program. It should include information about your child's current educational performance, goals and objectives for the next year, a statement about the services that will be provided, when those services will begin, and how your child's progress will be evaluated. Legally, your child's IEP must be reviewed and rewritten to keep up with changes in your child's needs at least once each year. An IEP meeting is held each year for this purpose.

If it has been established that your child will receive special education in any given school year, the IEP is supposed to be developed and in effect by the beginning (October 1) of the school year. If it is initially established that your child needs special education services after October 1, an IEP meeting must be held within 30 calendar days. The IEP meeting is often conducted in the spring in order to make plans for the new year. However, as long as the IEP is in effect by October 1 of the school year, agencies have flexibility about when they hold the meeting. In addition, if you are concerned about your child's IEP or about your child's program, you may request an IEP meeting at any time during the year.

A school system is responsible for implementing the IEP. They cannot refuse to implement the program or put your child on a waiting list because they do not have sufficient staff or a staff member who is trained to provide a particular service. They may arrange for someone outside of the school system to provide the service (for example, a private individual or another agency or school system). However, your child's school system is responsible for the costs of providing all services identified on the IEP.

The Individual Family Service Plan (IFSP). The IFSP is required in most states for children from birth through two years of age. A recent amendment to the legislation allows an IFSP to be done instead of an IEP for children from three to five if it is consistent with state policy. Thus an IFSP can be used at the discretion of the local education agency for children from three to five with the concurrence of the parents.

Services for children from birth through two years are provided by many different agencies. Therefore, the services identified on the IFSP may represent multiple providers. The law requiring services for children two and under is newer than the one requiring the services for older children (see Chapter 2 for more details). Most states have agreed to provide services to infants and toddlers. However, states are at slightly different stages in the process of planning and implementing the services. If you are not sure if your state has committed to providing services to children under three, call the lead agency or State Education agency listed in the appendix of this book for your state. The lead agency is the agency in your state which has the responsibility for overseeing services to children under three years of age.

As the name suggests, the IFSP is a somewhat different document than the IEP. The most important difference is that the IFSP and the services that are provided should focus on your entire family rather than only on your child. The IFSP must include information about your child's present levels of physical development, cognitive development, language and speech development, psychosocial development and self-help skills. In addition, the IFSP must include a statement of your family's concerns, priorities and resources as they relate to enhancing your child's development. The IFSP must also include a statement of major outcomes expected for your child and family, and provide specific information as to how those outcomes are to be achieved. It must provide a statement of the specific services necessary to meet the needs of your child and of your family (as they may relate to enhancing your child's development), the frequency, intensity and location of the services; payment arrangements (if any) and a description of appropriate time-lines. In addition, the IFSP must include a description of the steps that will be taken to move your child to a preschool program when he or she is three. A service coordinator who is in charge of coordinating all the services and implementing the plan must be identified. Finally, to the extent that it is appropriate, the IFSP must also identify medical and other services that your child needs (other than routine medical services). However, it is important to realize that although these "other services" are listed, they are not entitlements and there may be costs associated with them. They are listed in order to help provide a comprehensive picture of your child's needs. If necessary, the IFSP should include the steps that will be undertaken to help you obtain the services through private or public resources. Part of the service coordinator's role is to help you obtain these services if necessary. The IFSP is to be reviewed twice per year. The initial IFSP should be developed within 45 days of your child's first referral. It is reviewed every six months. It can be reviewed more frequently if circumstances require it or if you request a review.

At this point, you may be wondering why there are such differences between the IEP and the IFSP. For the most part, these differences exist because the types of services that are needed by infants and toddlers are often quite different from those needed by older children. For example, programs for infants and toddlers often take place at home rather than in a center the way that preschool programs do. Also, the laws reflect changes in the central role of the family for children's development.

Requirements for the IEP and IFSP Meeting

IEP or IFSP meetings are designed to assure that parents have a chance to give their opinions about the services that are provided for their child. The purpose is for parents and professionals to work *together* to make decisions about the most appropriate services. The law intends for you to be an equal part of the team.

- Legally, the meeting must be scheduled at a place and a time that is convenient for you.

- The meeting must be held in your native language (or other mode of communication) or provide an interpreter provided it is clearly not feasible.

- You must be informed of the purpose, time, and place of the meeting in time to attend.

- The school or program should also let you know the names of all participants and

- you may invite other people.

At IEP meetings, the school system must make sure that the following people are present: one or both parents, the child's teacher, and a school system or agency representative who is authorized to commit resources and make decisions about the services the agency will provide (for example, an administrator or school principal). In addition, if this is your child's first IEP meeting, the person who evaluated the child or someone who is familiar with the evaluation results must also be present. Other personnel are also present in many instances if they have information that is likely to have some bearing on the IEP. In addition, *you* may invite other people (e.g, friends, an advocate, an outside professional who is familiar with your child's needs) to attend the meeting. You can also include your child, although this is most often done with older students. Not all persons who work with your child are required to attend the meeting. However, if there is a professional who you consider critical to your child's program (for example, a therapist or vision teacher) by all means request that the person attend. If your child has been evaluated for the first time, the meeting must also include a member of the evaluation team and someone else (for example, your child's teacher) who is familiar with the evaluation procedures and the results. The school or agency is required to inform you who will attend the meeting.

IFSP meetings are very similar in the way they are constructed. The following persons should be present: one or both parents; other family members if you request their presence and it is feasible; an advocate or person outside of the family if you request it; the service coordinator; a person (or persons) directly involved in evaluating or assessing your child and, as appropriate, persons who will be providing services to the child and family. If, for some reason, one of these persons cannot attend, the program must make arrangements for their involvement through other means (such as having their representative attend the meeting, having a telephone conference or making relevant records available).

Given the family-centered focus of the IFSP, more attention may be given to family needs in IFSP meetings than in IEP meetings.

Benefits of the IEP and IFSP Meetings

IEP and IFSP meetings provide many opportunities for parents. The meetings give you a chance to personally meet the service providers who are directly involved in your child's program. It is a great opportunity to clear up points of confusion. For example, professionals on your child's team will sometimes have different opinions about some aspect of your child's behavior or development. This may be a good chance to have everyone resolve such differences in opinion. In addition, the meeting will force everyone to see the "total picture". One parent told us that "...with the physical therapist working on motor development and the speech therapist working on communication and the teacher on cognitive skills, I felt that everyone saw my child as just a bunch of little pieces". When together in one room, everyone is forced to look at the effect of each service provider's goals on other parts of your child's program.

In addition to the benefits of bringing together a large number of individuals who provide services for your child and family, IEP and IFSP meetings offer other opportunities for parents as well. At this meeting, you can learn about your child's progress. It is an opportunity to share information with service providers that may be significant in your child's development. It is also an opportunity to identify additional needs that your child and your family may have. If you have obtained individual evaluations, you can share the results and use the information to advocate for a change in the services your child is receiving. As you add information to the service providers' observations, goals can be changed and placement decisions discussed and altered. You can also use this time as an opportunity to clarify or resolve differences you may have regarding your child's educational program.

Concerns Parents Have Expressed About the Meetings

Despite the potential benefits of IEP/IFSP meetings, many parents find themselves feeling a little anxious or uncomfortable as the meeting approaches. If this has happened to you, you are certainly not alone! There are many reasons you may feel this way. One reason is that there are sometimes a large number of professionals at the meeting. This can happen because there are frequently many people who are directly involved in the services that are provided for a particular child and family. Each one of them will have some information to contribute. Although it is important to have this information, it is not uncommon to feel a little overwhelmed by the number of people you are meeting and the amount of information you are receiving. Second, since school systems often have numerous IEP and IFSP meetings to conduct, you may feel rushed or that you have not had a chance to discuss your concerns. Another problem is that professionals may refer to assessment information which is new to you or which you do not understand. Some parents have complained at times that not all of the professionals who are important to their child's program are at the meeting. Still others have reported feeling that the important decisions have already been made and that professionals just want parents to sign the document and leave.

If any of these situations have occurred for you, try to keep several things in mind.

- First, try to take some comfort in knowing that you are not alone. Many parents have reported such feelings.

- Second, professionals certainly do not intend for you to have this experience. It is often the outgrowth of trying to meet the needs of many different children and their families or of working within service systems that are bureaucratic.

- Third, there are some things that you can do to prepare yourself for the meeting and things you can do in the meeting to make sure that the needs of your child and your family are addressed.

- Finally, keep in mind that these meetings can often be difficult emotionally even when things go well. One mother said

> "Even when I get all of the services I want for my son, I never fail to leave the meetings with a lump in my throat. It is still so hard to hear about all of the things he *can't* do that other children his age can do."

Preparing for the Meeting

Taking a little time before the meeting to prepare can be a big help in reducing any nervousness you may feel. Even if you don't feel anxious, you will probably find that a little bit of preparation can go a long way in helping you obtain the services you want for your child. Several strategies may help you prepare.

1) Spend some time thinking about what you believe your child's strengths and needs are. To do this ask yourself some questions.

- What can your child *already* do (e.g., sit up, hold a bottle, listen to sounds, smile, etc)?
- What do *you* hope that (s)he will learn in the next year?
- What are your child's likes and dislikes, (e.g. does he love music, have a favorite toy, have favorite foods)?

Table 7-1
Preparing for the Meeting

- THINK ABOUT YOUR CHILD'S STRENGTHS AND NEEDS
- WRITE DOWN ANY GOALS, OBJECTIVES OR OUTCOMES THAT ARE IMPORTANT TO YOU
- THINK ABOUT YOUR FAMILY'S CONCERNS, PRIORITIES AND RESOURCES
- WRITE DOWN YOUR QUESTIONS ABOUT YOUR CHILD'S PROGRAM
- DECIDE IF YOU WANT SOMEONE WITH YOU AT THE MEETING
- OBSERVE YOUR CHILD'S CURRENT OR FUTURE PLACEMENT
- IF NECESSARY, OBTAIN AN OUTSIDE ASSESSMENT
- DRESS SO THAT YOU WILL BE COMFORTABLE WITH THE SERVICE PROVIDERS
- BRING RELEVANT FILES AND OTHER DOCUMENTATION TO THE MEETING
- LET THE SCHOOL KNOW IF YOU CAN'T ATTEND DUE TO PROBLEMS WITH TRANSPORTATION, CHILD CARE OR A TIME CONFLICT

- Are there special ways your child uses to tell you these things (e.g., does he always laugh when a certain song is on the radio; does he always refuse certain foods)?

By answering these questions for yourself ahead of time, you will have a better idea about whether your goals and the service providers' goals are the same. For example, you may think that your child should be around children without disabilities, have a way to communicate, be toilet trained, or wish that he could feed himself. Remember, you are likely to have more answers to some of these questions than the service providers. For example, information about your child's likes and dislikes and the ways that he communicates with you may be very helpful to professionals who do not yet know your child.

Take a few minutes to jot down the answers to these questions. That way, when you go to the meeting, you can make sure that the information that you have to offer about your child is incorporated and that your goals for your child are addressed.

You may find that it is easier to keep track of the information described in your notes if you keep a single notebook in which you write these questions down as they come up. Then, when the time for the meeting arrives, you can take out your list.

(2) If you are attending an IFSP meeting, go through the same process for your family's concerns, priorities and resources as they relate to your child. What would be most helpful to your family (e.g., having your child sleep through the night, giving him/her a way to communicate, getting some trained respite care, finding a support group)? Even if you are attending an IEP meeting rather than an IFSP meeting, thinking about your family's needs will help you maintain a broad perspective. You may even find that the school has opportunities to help you address these needs (e.g., such as parent support groups) that you were not aware of.

(3) Write down the questions that you have about your child and his or her program. Your questions might include such things as the meaning of certain terms that are used, confusion over information that seems to conflict with other information you have received, questions about future placements and so forth.

(4) Decide if you want to take someone with you to the meeting. You have the right to bring anyone you wish. The person can be anyone you choose

including another family member or a good friend. It can also be another service provider who has worked with your child in another capacity and who is willing to come to the meeting to offer support and/or provide additional information. Taking someone else to the meeting will give you someone with whom you can share your impressions and concerns after the meeting. This is especially helpful if you are single or if your spouse is unable to attend. Inform the program ahead of time that someone else will be coming.

(5) Consider observing your child's current placement or a future placement before your meeting. Observing the placement will be especially helpful if your child is in a center-based program and you have not yet visited the classroom. This will give you the opportunity to observe your child, learn your child's routine, and get to know the program staff. All children, with or without disabilities, act differently in different environments, but you may be surprised to see your own child doing things she is unwilling to attempt at home or refusing to do things that you know she can do well.

Observing a future placement is also advisable if it is time for your child to change placements (e.g., from a home-based to a center-based setting). This will give you a chance to predict what your child will encounter in a new setting and raise questions that you want answered before you agree to a new placement. If you are unsure if it is time for a new placement ask your child's teacher or another service provider before the meeting. You can also find out how to arrange an observation of potential placements so that you will be prepared for the meeting.

When you observe the potential placement site, observe the way in which the teacher interacts with other children, how the environment is arranged, and how behavior is managed to make sure the teacher's approach is consistent with your own viewpoints. Try to envision your child's reactions to these factors. Talk to the teacher and ask any questions you may have. For example, if your child is about to move into a regular preschool or kindergarten, find out if the teacher has had other children with disabilities in her classroom before. You may want to find out if she uses any special techniques to prepare the nondisabled children for the presence of a child with a disability. You might even volunteer to participate in such an orientation of your child's classmates, explaining such things as the way your child communicates or what her special likes and dislikes are. Again, write your reactions, thoughts, questions and concerns in your notebook as a reference for the meeting.

(6) If necessary, obtain an outside assessment. If you have reason to believe that your views will be challenged or if you already know you have serious disagreements with one or more of the professionals on your child's team, consider obtaining an outside evaluation. This will enable you to document your viewpoint during the meeting. However, it is wise to find out whether you will be responsible for the costs of such an evaluation before you proceed.

(7) Dress in a way that makes you feel comfortable with the professionals who will be present. This will vary depending on the size and formality of the program. Although there are certainly no dress requirements, you may feel intimidated or uncomfortable if all of the service providers are dressed up and you are not.

(8) Bring your portable file system with you to the meeting (see Chapter 4, Managing the Information). If your system is not portable, or is too cumbersome, pull any pieces of information (e.g., reports from specialists) that have accumulated since your last meeting and take them to the meeting. You will be able to refer to the documents if necessary. This is especially important if the program does not have the new information or if you need to document a point you want to make during the meeting. You may also want to take the last IEP or IFSP so you can determine if previous objectives or outcomes were accomplished.

(9) If you have difficulty attending the meeting for some reason such as a transportation problem, child care for other children, or time conflict, be sure to let the school know. Make it clear that you want to come to the meeting. If your problem is transportation, the program may be able to help you with school or van transportation or be able to provide a taxi voucher. Remember, the program must reschedule the meeting if you wish to be there and cannot attend at the scheduled time.

AT THE MEETING

You will probably meet in an office, library or meeting room around a table or a desk. Depending on how many people work with your child, there may be as few as two people. However it is not unusual to have many more than this. Five to seven people is not uncommon and we have heard stories of meetings including as many as twenty people. One person will probably coordinate the meeting. If you are introduced to many new people at once, make an effort to write down the name and position of each person. One idea is to take name tags and ask each person

---

Table 7-2
Tips for the Meeting

- MAKE SURE YOU ARE INTRODUCED

- HAVE SERVICE PROVIDERS WEAR NAME TAGS OR WRITE DOWN THEIR NAME AND POSITION

- INTRODUCE ANYONE YOU HAVE BROUGHT TO THE MEETING

- TAKE A TAPE RECORDER

- MAKE IT CLEAR HOW YOU WISH TO BE ADDRESSED

- TRY TO STAY CALM AND EVEN-TEMPERED

- GET SPECIFIC INFORMATION ON THE ASSESSMENT PROCEDURES USED

- MAKE SURE YOUR CHILD'S STRENGTHS ARE AC-KNOWLEDGED

- MAKE SURE PROFESSIONALS ADDRESS YOUR PRIORI-TIES FOR YOUR CHILD AND FAMILY

- ASK PROFESSIONALS TO CLARIFY TERMS OR POINTS YOU DON'T UNDERSTAND

- RECOGNIZE THAT YOU HAVE KNOWLEDGE THAT PRO-FESSIONALS DO NOT

- STATE YOUR PREFERENCES ABOUT PLACEMENT DECI-SIONS

- IF TIME RUNS OUT TOO SOON, ASK FOR ANOTHER MEETING

- SIGN THE DOCUMENT ONLY IF YOU FEEL COMFORT-ABLE WITH THE PLAN.

- WORK CONSTRUCTIVELY WITH THE PROGRAM TO RE-SOLVE ANY DIFFERENCES

to put on a name tag with their name and position so that you know who is talking. If you don't know the professionals and they don't introduce themselves, stop the meeting and ask to be introduced. After all, this is your child and you have the right to know who is making recommendations about his program. If you don't insist on finding out who is present and what each person does, you may find yourself in the middle of the meeting and unable to tell who is talking and what their role is in your child's program.

This is also a good point to introduce anyone that you have brought to the meeting. Explain why you have asked them to attend (e.g, a source of outside information, moral support, etc) and what their role will be in the meeting.

At the beginning of the meeting, clarify how much time is available, and find out whether everyone will be staying for the entire meeting. This way you can make certain that key persons will be present during the discussion of special issues and that there is enough time to devote to issues that are of special importance to you.

If you are afraid the meeting will move too quickly for you, think about taking a tape recorder. A tape will allow you to go back later and listen to what was said. You can listen to the tape later if you forget something or were unclear during the meeting. If you must attend alone, this will give your spouse and other interested parties the opportunity to hear what was said directly and save you from having to explain something that you were not clear about. Be sure to tell everyone at the beginning of the meeting that you will be taping it. If you are not taping the meeting and it goes too fast for you, do not be afraid to ask whoever is talking to slow down enough for you to take notes. (Note: If the agency tapes the meeting, it is considered an educational record and is confidential.)

If some of the professionals address you as "mom" or "dad" and you do not feel comfortable with this, tell them so and indicate how you would like to be addressed. This can be done in a positive manner such as "Feel free to call me George" or "I like to be called Mrs. Brown".

At the beginning of the meeting each specialist will probably review the assessments in their area of expertise. Have each service provider specify which tests were administered and the results of each one. You can ask for a copy of the test results if you wish to do so for your files. Having copies of these records can be important later on. Even if you feel that you will not understand the results, other professionals may be able to learn valuable information from the tests or reports at another time.

- If you are unsure of what specific test results mean for your child's intervention program, ask the professionals involved to clarify this information.

- If you don't agree with the evaluation results, make this clear and give your reasons.

- If the service provider says that your child was not able to do certain things that you have seen him/her do, give examples of what you have seen at home. Young children frequently do things at home that they do not do in a test situation. The service providers should be grateful for the information and may be able to incorporate the information you provide.

- If that is not possible, find out how much the particular item with which you disagree will affect your child's program (either in terms of intervention goals or placements).

- If you still disagree and the item has a strong impact on plans for your child, you can ask for an independent evaluation. The requirements governing the IEP state that parents have a right to an independent evaluation (sometimes at public expense). Although the same provision is technically not part of the federal requirements governing the IFSP, some states apply the same rules. Even if your state does not, there is reason to believe that you could offer the results of such an evaluation at a due process hearing (see Chapter 9, Due Process) if your disagreement goes that far (Turnbull & Turnbull, 1991).

- If there are lengthy written assessment reports which you do not have time to read while you are listening to people speak, focus for the time on the conversation. Remember, you can read the reports more carefully at home and telephone back for additional information or to question results.

On the IFSP, there will be a place to identify the concerns, priorities and resources of your family. Hopefully, these will be identified through ongoing interviews with you.

- If you feel that your child or family has strengths or resources that have not been captured, speak up! It is important that the professionals involved notice these resources and strengths in order to form the most positive view of you and your family. Moreover, these resources and strengths are a solid foundation around which everyone can build.

- This is also the point to discuss any priorities and concerns that your family may have as they relate to your child. For example, if you really need to find someone who can stay with your child when you are away, this is a good time to bring it up. If you and your family are desperate to have your child sleep through the night, this is a legitimate family concern. Identify anything that would help you cope.

- At some point, both the IEP and the IFSP meeting will focus on the program and services which are to be provided for your child. If you are in an IFSP meeting, professionals may refer to "child outcomes". If you are in an IEP meeting, professionals will refer to "goals" and "objectives". **When the meeting reaches this point, be sure to let the professionals know which areas are of high priority to you.**

- If you disagree with the outcomes, goals and/or objectives that are stated, ask the professional to explain the importance and purpose. Explain why you disagree, providing as many examples as possible.

- Find out how progress will be measured and who will be responsible for working on a particular goal, outcome, or objective.

As the meeting proceeds, individual professionals may use words, expressions or talk about equipment that you do not understand. If this happens, stop whoever is talking and ask for a clear explanation. In addition, professionals may make suggestions or give you things to do with your child that you don't understand. Remember, this is most often *not* your fault. Often, service providers get so used to using a particular technique or professional jargon that they forget that most people are not familiar with it. Just let the service provider know that you need further explanation. For example, a physical therapist may offer suggestions for working with your child at home which are confusing. Even if you are given diagrams, the procedure may seem unclear. Ask for clarification or if necessary, set up an appointment to come to a physical therapy session so that you can learn these techniques well. Most therapists and teachers care very genuinely for the children with whom they work and will be glad for your expression of interest. Keep in mind that they may also find it frustrating not to be able to communicate their suggestions more clearly.

On the other hand, sometimes professionals may assume that you understand much less than you do. They need to hear that their preceptions are
incorrect. For example, if your child is fragile medically, you have probably been responsible for some complicated home medical care before
your child ever enters a center-based program. In all likelihood, you have
information and experience with your child that teachers can learn from.
If your child is using respiratory equipment or is tube fed or has a medical
condition requiring extensive treatment, you may be able to explain to
educational professionals about the ways that this affects his alertness,
behavior, or moods. You may also have to show them how to use some
of this equipment or arrange a training session for them with a doctor or
nurse.

After the teacher or therapist has suggested goals and objectives for
your child, ask yourself if you have seen your child engage in the desired
behavior at home. If so, tell the service providers.

- If there are goals which you feel your child is ready to move
  toward but which are not listed, mention those as well.

- Bring up expectations or needs of family members which relate
  to the issues being discussed.

- If you have questions or disagree with the goals, objectives or
  outcomes, it is important to bring up those questions.

- If the professional feels that your child is not ready yet for
  something that you would like to see as a goal, listen carefully to
  their explanations and see if these match your perceptions of your
  child's skills and potential.

- Also, look over your notes from home to be sure your child does
  not have medical or other special needs which should be addressed.

- Listen carefully to the interventionists' responses to your questions. You may want to jot notes for yourself if you are not taping
  the meeting.

At some point during the meeting there will be a discussion of the most
appropriate placement for your child. This is a critical point because it
will determine your child's program for the upcoming six months to one
year.

If you have preferences, this is the time to state them. For example, if it is important to you that your child be fully included in a regular preschool program or daycare center, *say so!* If you feel your child would benefit by moving from a home-based infant program to a center-based program for toddlers or preschool children, let everyone know. If you have not had an opportunity to observe a potential new placement and you feel uncertain about it, tell everyone that you want a chance to observe before you make a commitment. This is also the time to make sure that your child is getting all of the other services (See Chapter 3, Working with Multiple Service Providers for more information on placements and other services).

If time is short and you feel that there is a lot of unfinished business, ask for a second meeting. You should also consider asking for a follow-up meeting if certain key professionals are unable to attend and you want their input.

By the end of the meeting, you will be asked to sign the IEP or IFSP document. If you feel comfortable with the plan you should, by all means, sign the document.

However, if you feel unhappy with the plan or feel that too much remains unsettled, *you are not required to sign it.* Agencies typically want signatures because it is a way for the program to document attendance and is a way to document that you approved of your child's program. As a result, agencies are usually eager to work with you so that you will feel comfortable enough to sign the document. It may be necessary to hold an additional meeting in order to obtain agreement. If your efforts to resolve the disagreement are not successful, you may want to consider asking for mediation or exercising your right to an impartial due process hearing. At this point you should ask for information about the guidelines for a due process hearing or any alternative mediation procedures (see Chapter 9 for more detailed information on this process). If at any point, you are uncertain about your legal rights, ask for clarification.

AFTER THE MEETING

When the meeting is over, it is usually a good idea to reread the IEP or IFSP document slowly. You may need to call back to ask for more explanation of points that you don't recall or don't understand. You may also think of additional information that you believe should be included.

For example, if your child has made little progress in physical therapy over the last six months but has spent two of those months recovering from major illness or surgery, you may want that information reflected in the therapist's report.

If your questions and concerns remain unanswered, you may want to request either another informal meeting or another IEP or IFSP meeting. This is especially true if your concerns are serious and affect your child's program, the quality of your child's life or your family in some way.

If you are unhappy about the outcome of the meeting, you can request mediation (in some states) or a due process hearing. You can also request an outside evaluation by a psychologist, developmental evaluation clinic or other specialist. If you have serious concerns that your child has not been accurately diagnosed and/or is not receiving the services that he or she needs, an outside evaluation may be an important source of information. For example, the report of an orthopedic physician or an outside therapist can provide outside documentation of the need for physical or occupational therapy.

Some children, as a result of early intervention, are able to progress to regular preschool and kindergarten classes with other children who do not have disabilities. You may need an outside evaluation to assure that this progress is well-documented and that your child is not mislabeled as he or she enters public school.

At other times, children test well in early intervention but their parents have an underlying fear that there is something wrong or that there may be a serious, unrecognized problem which might influence school progress. This too may need documentation by a specialist in the area of concern. Your pediatrician or your child's program may be able to help you find the best resources in your area and may be able to give you a referral. Other sources of information are provided in the list of resources for each state that are provided in the appendix. Be sure to clarify who is responsible for the costs of such an evaluation.

BETWEEN MEETINGS

Many issues are likely to arise between meetings. Notice how your child is progressing toward the goals identified in the IEP or IFSP. Many different patterns of developmental progress be seen. Some children seem to make steady progress which may seem relatively insignificant at the time but which is very significant over a three- or six-month period. Other children go through periods where they make breakthroughs developmentally and through periods where it seems as if they are not making much progress. It may help to think back to how your child was doing over the holidays or last summer and see what progress you notice toward his or her goals. If something significant happens at home, let the school or intervention program know so that they can watch for the same things and modify day to day objectives for your child accordingly.

If your child has major medical problems, be sure these are communicated to the school or service provider, even if you don't think they will affect the program. Such problems can influence your child's alertness, fussiness and general performance. For example, if your child is taking seizure medications and there is a change in dosage or type of medication, this may have an influence on his or her behavior. In some cases, serious medical problems may influence the skills your child is able to demonstrate. You may want to have information about a medical setback or recovery recorded in your child's record.

If something is going on at home that could influence your child's performance or behavior, it may be important to let the school or service provider know. For example, some young children have difficulty adjusting to the birth of a baby brother or sister. It may help the teacher to know that your child is making such an adjustment. Moreover, since this is such a normal part of growing up, your teacher may have ideas about ways you can help this adjustment process along. If your family is preparing for a move that will affect your child's daily routine or her school placement, it will help to let the school know. They can help by preparing or updating reports to be sent or taken to a new center. They may be able to refer you to programs in your area and help you identify especially good programs. It is also possible that one of the professionals you are working with will have professional contacts in the new location that can assist you on your arrival.

CONCLUSION

The IEP and IFSP meetings are an important part of your child's intervention program. It is easy to feel intimidated by the amount of information and by the many professionals involved. Remember that this is *your* child and your family. You have information to offer that is as important as that of the service providers and legitimate ideas about the needs of your child and your family. We hope that the tips we have provided here can help clear up some of the confusion and help you gain confidence about advocating effectively in these meetings.

CHAPTER 8

Handling Transitions

Susan A. Fowler and Patricia F. Titus

You and your child will start and leave services several times during the first five years of your child's life. The transition from one service program to another program can be both a positive and a challenging experience. Typically your family is leaving something familiar and starting something new. To some extent, each change in programs represents the passage of a milestone for your family. Your child is growing and acquiring new skills. You are learning to negotiate a new service system. In this chapter we will address the issues of moving from an early intervention program to preschool, moving from preschool to elementary school, and changing programs due to family moves.

Each transition will require you to gather information, make decisions, and take the risk that you and your child can adjust to and benefit from the new program. Some transitions mark a cause for celebration for your child's development, some may mark a moment of sadness for development that has not occurred yet. And leaving behind a program and staff whom you have come to trust and rely on can be difficult.

There are several important points to remember about transition. They are a part of life — everyone experiences changes in programs. Successful transitions between programs usually require planning and communication between the family and the program staff. Information exchanges and planning between the staff of the sending and receiving programs also must occur. Parents and staff will need time to communicate if they are to share information, ask questions, make recommendations and broach concerns. The development of trust between parents and the new receiving program often will depend on the time allowed to share information, to visit and observe the new program, and the tone or receptivity of the program staff to family issues.

As the parent and primary care provider for your child, you have a right to participate in the decisions regarding any change in your child's program. You can play several roles in the process and you can determine the extent to which you wish to be involved. At the very least, you should be kept informed of the process.

THE TRANSITION FROM AN EARLY INTERVENTION PROGRAM TO A PRESCHOOL PROGRAM

Many families with infants and toddlers who have disabilities or who are developmentally delayed will receive early intervention services. These services may be provided in your home; if your child attends a day care program, they may be provided there. In some instances, early intervention services are provided in a center or clinic. The transition from early intervention services to preschool services will occur on or near your child's third birthday. In many cases this transition will involve movement to a center-based program. Typically the special education and related services provided within the preschool program will be associated with the local public schools. Table 8-1 presents the federal regulations that support transition planning for your child. These rules apply to every state. These regulations help assure that your child moves from the early intervention program to a preschool program without disrupting or losing necessary services. This means that you *should not have to wait for a new program and you should be involved in discussions regarding future placements.*

What are the steps involved in this transition? Every family will have their own set of questions and needs and families will differ in the extent to which they choose to be involved in transition planning and decision-making. So the number of steps a family takes in moving from one program to another will vary. Seven steps that many families take are listed below.

Attend a planning meeting.

At least ninety days prior to your child's third birthday, your individualized family service plan (IFSP) must be amended to include plans for facilitating the transition. You should be invited to a meeting at this time to: (a) discuss your child's progress; (b) provide consent for staff to contact the local education agency to release information about your child; (c) review your child's program options, and; (d) establish a plan for transition activities. As you can see in Table 8-1, federal regulations

Table 8-1
Individuals with Disabilities Act Amendments of 1991
(Reauthorization P.L.102-119)

Part H
  Section 303.344 "Content of the IFSP"
  Subsection (h)

(h) Transition at age three.

  (1) The IFSP must include the steps to be taken to support the transition of the child, upon reaching age three, to—

   (i) Preschool services under Part B of the Act, to the extent that those services are considered appropriate; or

   (ii) Other services that may be available, if appropriate.

  (2) The steps required in paragraph (h) (1) of this section include—

   (i) Discussions with, and training of, parents regarding future placement and other matters related to the child's transition;

   (ii) Procedures to prepare the child for changes in services delivery, including steps to help the child adjust to, and function in, a new setting; and

   (iii) With parental consent, the transmission of information about the child to the local education agency, to ensure continuity of services, including evaluation and assessment information required in 303.322, and copies of IFSPs that have been developed and implemented in accordance with 303.340 and 303.346.

Source: U.S.Department of Education, 34 CFR Part 303: Early intervention programs for infants and toddlers with handicaps. *Federal Register.* June 22, 1989; Vol.54: 26322

require that all early intervention programs begin discussions with families about transition at least three months before children turn 3 years of age. It often takes this much time to complete all the necessary planning for a smooth transition. You should remind the staff to schedule the meeting, if they have not mentioned it to you.

Discuss your child's progress. This meeting provides an opportunity for you to discuss your child's progress. It also is a time to identify your preferences and concerns regarding the next services for your child. Questions often asked by families include: Has my child progressed at the rate we expected? Is my child ready for a new program? Can my child continue in this program longer (or until the end of the school year)? What can I do to prepare my child for the change in programs? Will my child ride a bus to the new school? Is the bus safe? What are my program choices? Will the new teacher know about and like my child? Will my child know any of the children in the new class?

The program staff should be sensitive to the range of questions that you may have. It may not be possible to address or answer all of these questions at the initial planning meeting. However, finding answers to the questions can become a part of the transition plan; so can providing time and the opportunity for you to ask these questions of staff at programs that may serve their child. Parents whose children have completed the transitions also are a valuable resource for parents just facing the change of programs.

Discuss parent consent for the release of information about your child to the local education agency. Your written consent must be obtained before staff at the early intervention program contacts the public schools or transmits information about your child to the next program. Parents have a right to review and approve all information that is sent to the next program. You should ask the staff for your child's file and review the materials that the staff recommends be forwarded to the public schools. Usually, the results of screening tests, developmental assessments, recent evaluation reports, eligibility determinations for continued services, and copies of the Individualized Family Service Plan are forwarded. According to the law, you have the right to review these records and any other records that involve your child and your family. The agency must comply with your request "without unnecessary delay" and at most within two weeks (note to 34 CFR 303.423).

If you agree with the information and give consent for it to be released, the service coordinator from the early intervention program will share assessment information and the IFSP with appropriate staff from the local education agency. This information is often helpful in ensuring continuity in services for your child. The preschool program should be able to build on this information and begin services at the level at which the early intervention services ended.

On rare occasions, a family may have concerns about information contained in their child's report. Legal safeguards have been developed to protect your rights to privacy and accuracy. You should feel free to discuss your concerns about the records with the staff. They should respond to reasonable requests for explanations and interpretations of the record and provide you with a copy of the record.

If you think that the information in your child's file is inaccurate or misleading or violates the privacy of your family, you are entitled to request that the information be amended or deleted. (See 34 CFR, 300. 567-300. 570.) If you make this request, the agency staff must act on it within 45 days.

If the staff refuses to amend the information as requested, they must inform you and advise you that you may resolve the complaint through a complaint resolution process. (See 34. CFR 303.420).

If you choose not to appeal or lose the appeal, you have the right to place a statement in your child's file commenting on the information that you consider misleading or invasive.

Discuss your child's eligibility for continued special education services.
It is important to determine if your child will continue to need special services. Preschool special education and related services are administered by the local public schools in most states. This means that the program staff from the early intervention program or the public school should provide you with information regarding the eligibility criteria for special education preschool services in your state. They should discuss with you whether your child's current developmental level appears to meet those criteria. If you and the early intervention staff are not sure that your child qualifies for continued special services, you should discuss what evaluations and assessments are needed to determine your child's eligibility for continued services during the planning meeting. You should also identify who is going to provide the assessments. The early intervention program and your local public school program should know who conducts these assessments and which agency is financially responsible for the evaluation. These assessments should be scheduled

soon after this meeting so that there is enough time to determine your child's eligibility and to choose the most appropriate services. You should be informed of the assessment results as soon as they are available. Some states require that children who are eligible for preschool services receive a diagnostic label that categorizes their disability, such as mentally retarded, or speech and language impaired. In other states, children who qualify will be identified only as developmentally delayed, until age 6. You should ask if your child will receive a specific label.

Review your child's program options. Some children who receive early intervention will no longer need special education and related services. For instance, a child may not demonstrate the delays at age 3 that were evident at age 1. Other children may not qualify for continued services at age 3 because their delays are not substantial enough for them to meet the eligibility criteria for preschool special education services. For instance, in some states children who exhibit a mild delay in one area, may not qualify for services because the state's criteria for eligibility requires evidence of a delay in two areas or a severe delay in one area. In these cases, the IFSP should contain steps to assist families who want continued services, to identify and find other services for their child. Such services may include public programs such as Head Start or private programs such as community preschools.

If your child continues to be eligible for special education services, the transition plan should contain steps for identifying free, appropriate services which provide special education. Such programs must be provided in the least restrictive environment. This means that your child should receive services which best meet his or her individual needs and which are provided in settings in which children without disabilities also are served. The program options may include: (a) special education preschools located in neighborhood public schools; (b) integrated community preschools in which special education services are provided; or (c) co-enrollment in a special education preschool which serves only children with disabilities and in a second program which serves children without disabilities. Some school districts provide all three options; others provide one or two of these options.

Develop the transition plan

The transition plan in the IFSP should be developed in the planning meeting based on the initial information that is shared. The plan should be flexible so that it can be revised as additional information is obtained. Table 8-2 contains a sample transition plan for a family whose daughter's eligibility for preschool services had not been determined prior to the initial planning meeting and whose family wished to consider private program options as well as the special education preschool in the local public school.

At a minimum, the transition plan should include the following steps: (a) discussions with parents regarding future placements and their rights to receive services; (b) procedures to prepare the child for changes in service delivery; (c) with parent consent, the transfer of information about the child, including evaluation and assessment information and copies of the IFSP to the next program.

Include steps for discussions with parents. The initial planning meeting and the transition plan should provide parents with a picture of the transition process and options for their participation. Parents should be informed of the time frame for making decisions about their child's next program. They should know the steps involved in making a decision regarding the next program. They should be provided with the time and opportunity to determine their level of involvement in the steps. To enable you to choose your level of participation, you may wish to request a calendar of events or timeline to guide their involvement in the process. Table 8-3 presents an example of a timeline.

Other issues to discuss with program staff include the way changes in service delivery may affect your family. For instance, when children move from a home based program to a center based program, families often lose the frequent and consistent face-to-face contact with the service provider. If you wish to communicate as frequently with the new program staff, then you will need to discuss ways to do so. Options may include daily home notes, scheduled phone calls or scheduled or drop-in visits at the program. The change in frequency of contact may be a cause of concern or complaint by families, but one which can be avoided and understood through planning.

Include procedures to prepare your child for changes in services. Initiating the planning process 90 days prior to the child's birthday allows family and staff to plan how best to prepare the child for the next program. To some extent these plans may hinge upon the service delivery model selected for the next program.

The most typical transitions will involve: a) moving from a home-

Table 8-2
Family Transition Plan

Date: 3/1/91
Child's Name: L. J. Donovan
Date of Birth: 6/7/88

Goals	Strategies/Responsibilities	Timeline	Comments
1. EI Staff will coordinate evaluation of Laura with School District	Ms. Leahr (EI), Ms. Coleman (Schools), assess at home, by:	4/15	
2. Mrs. D will visit Rocking Horse Preschool, Learning Tree Preschool and public school Early Choices special education program to identify philosophy, routines, special services, family involvement, transportation options.	Ms. C will contact programs and visit by:	5/1	
3. Ms. L will assist family in forming a small play group for Laura. Will recommend strategies, activities, materials.	tip sheet, assist with 1st group by:	4/1	
4. Family will work with Laura on independence skills such as	assist family during home visits	3/6-6/6	
• reduce her use of pacifier outside of nap and bedtime	Use daily chart to record progress and prompt rewards for not using pacifier; start by:	3/6-	
• increase independence in taking coat on and off and hanging it up	tip sheet and practice during home visit; start by:	3/6-	
• pick up some toys daily before lunch and dinner	practice during home visit	4/15-	
• ignore frequent response of "no" to requests; praise compliance	practice during home visit	4/15-	
• practice saying first and last name in response to "what is your name"	practice during home visit	5/1-	

Table 8-3
A Sample Timeline for Planning the Transition from Early Intervention Services to Preschool Services

Laura Donovan's 3rd birthday: June 6

By March 6:	EI staff invite family to planning meeting to begin transition process.
By March 20	EI staff and family develop a transition plan.
By March 20	Family reviews Laura's records and provides consent for release of information to public school.
By April 15	EI and preschool staff identify necessary evaluations to determine eligibility for continued services and conduct evaluations.
By April 20	EI and preschool staff meet with family to discuss eligibility for continued services and to identify program options.
By May 1	Family and E.I. staff visit several placement options.
By May 15	Family and staffs from E.I and preschool meet to determine placement.
By June 1	Family and Laura visit the new program and meet with the teacher and related service staff.
By June 1	EI program transfers records to preschool and EI coordinator meets with Laura's preschool teacher to exchange information.
By June 10	Laura starts preschool; parents ride bus with Laura on first day of summer school.
By July 1	Family meets with preschool staff to assess Laura's adjustment.

based early intervention program to a center-based preschool program; b) moving from a home-based program to a combined center- and home-based program; and c) moving from one center-based program to another center-based program.

The transition from a home-based program to a center-based program raises many questions for families and service providers. Significant differences typically exist between the two models.

Families and early intervention staff should consider ways to prepare the child for the change in services. Some of the preparation can become a part of the daily family routine; other preparation steps may take careful planning. Four changes that affect many children when they first start a center-based program should be considered. They include: (a) separating from parents and home; (b) learning to play with peers and be part of a group; (c) following directions, routines and rules, and; (d) having safety skills.

Prepare the child for separation from family and home. This may be the child's first experience in which a parent or family member is not involved. To prepare their child for school separations, families may consider leaving their child at home with an experienced sitter for brief time periods so that both parent and child experience successful separations. These successful experiences in familiar surroundings may help the child learn that separations are temporary.

Prepare the child for group activities and peer play. You may wish to increase opportunities for your child to play in group settings and around other children. Informal strategies may include taking your child to parks with playground equipment where other children tend to play. You also might wish to invite children from the neighborhood to play. Again, these successful experiences may reduce the strangeness of entering a new program with a group of new children and a new teacher. If you are uncertain how to proceed, you may wish to discuss this with the early intervention providers and ask them to recommend groups or perhaps help to arrange a play group for your child.

Prepare the child for new routines and directions. Children may come into contact with new routines, rules and directions in a center program. Your child will benefit from experience in following directions and instructions prior to entry. Children sometimes experience difficulty if few demands have been placed on them at home to comply with instructions or if parents have been inconsistent in following through with children after giving an instruction. You may wish to practice simple routines at home (e.g., having your child hang his coat on a hook when he comes inside; asking your child to put her toys in a bin when finished playing) to familiarize your child with the fact that routines are a normal part of life. You may want to help your child practice following simple directions. This can be accomplished by playing games ("Simon says, stand up") and by using every day activities at home (e.g., "Find your shoes and socks").

Consider issues of child health and safety. Parents often are concerned about the safety of their child away from home, especially if this is their first transition to an out-of-home program. Issues to discuss and to prepare your child for may include: riding on the school bus or van and staying in the child safety seat; responding to the question, "what is your name" with first and last name (or wearing an identifying tag or label); asking for help.

Visit program options.

Some parents wish to visit the range of programs that are appropriate for their child. Other parents prefer not to do so, perhaps because of competing obligations and lack of time. The choice of the next program may be simple or complex, depending on the number of options considered and available. If your child is eligible for continued special education services, the public schools should provide you with information about the range of placements available for your child. You may also wish to consider private options and should feel free to visit those as well.

It is important to remember that the choice of program should be based on your *child's needs*. It should not be based on other factors, such as which program has an opening convenient to the time of transition. The IEP or the IFSP should identify the child's concerns, priorities and resources and the appropriate goals or outcomes. The selected placement should be one which is appropriate for achieving these goals or outcomes.

Attend the placement meeting.

Prior to your child's third birthday, a meeting should occur to select the next placement. This may be arranged by the early intervention program or by the local public school. At this meeting, several issues may be discussed.

- First, family and staff should determine whether the child is ready to make the transition on or near the third birthday. There is nothing magical about the third birthdate; it is simply a convenient way to ensure that children who are ready have access to special education preschool services. The option of remaining in early intervention services until the end of the school year can be discussed. This decision should be based on your child's needs and your child's readiness to enter a center-based program. If your child remains in the early intervention program until the end of the school year (e.g., May or June), it is the responsibility of the two agencies to determine which agency will be responsible for paying for the extension of the early intervention services. Your child should not be left without services.

- Second, if your child is ready to make the transition, then family and staff should determine which placement is most appropriate to the needs of the child. Families who have observed programs should share their observations and opinions at this time. More information on this process is provided in Chapter 7.

Visit the selected program with your child.

Once a placement is selected, it is often helpful to take your child on a planned visit to the program and to introduce her to the classroom and to the new staff. Sometimes it is helpful for the child first to visit the classroom when only the teachers are present so she can meet the teachers and explore the materials and equipment at her own pace. A second visit could be scheduled when other children are present and during an activity in which your child is likely to participate and enjoy (perhaps snack or a free play time). Such visits often help to reduce parental concerns about how their child fits in the new program. If the visits show that your child is having difficulty separating, you and the staff can develop a plan together for easing your child into the program. If a visit is not possible, you can help prepare your child for the transition by talking positively about the new school and the many new experiences and activities there.

Exchange information with the new staff about your child.

Many parents find that it is reassuring and helpful to share information with the new staff just before their child begins school or shortly afterwards. The family's perspective on the child's strengths and interests are very helpful to the staff. Discussions about what you can do or would like to do at home to support the child in the program are also helpful, as well as identifying strategies for communicating between home and school.

Maintain communication with the new program and expect the adjustment to take a little time.

Movement to a new program involves change and uncertainty for everyone. It is normal to be anxious about how your child adjusts and to want frequent reports from your child's new teacher. It helps if you have agreed upon a system of communicating and follow it. Daily or weekly notes are used by many programs for sharing information, especially when children ride the bus and parents cannot often visit the program.

Children often show adjustment stress too, particularly if they have not attended a day-care or preschool program before. They often are fussy and tired after school and this may continue for the first several weeks of preschool. It may take time for your child to build up endurance to everything new and become comfortable with the new routines. If you become concerned about your child's adjustment, you should discuss your concerns with the staff in the new program.

THE TRANSITION
FROM PRESCHOOL TO ELEMENTARY SCHOOL

Children typically leave preschool services between the age of five and six years and enter elementary school programs, usually a kindergarten class and in some cases, a special education program. There is no legal requirement that preschool programs begin a transition plan 90 days before the child's preschool program ends. However, developing a plan is considered best practice and you should ask your preschool to include a plan in your child's IEP or IFSP during the last year of preschool. The process should be very similar to the planning that you used in transitioning from the early intervention program to preschool. At least 90 days prior to the end of preschool you should request a meeting to discuss your child's progress and to identify program options. Critical questions to ask are:

1. What do recent evaluations tell us about my child's performance? Is my child performing within a normal developmental range for a five year-old?

2. If not, will my child receive support services in kindergarten? Is my child eligible for special education and related services?

3. How can we make sure that my child's services are not disrupted and that the kindergarten can build upon the services provided during preschool?

4. What are the options at the kindergarten level and which options will meet my child's needs best?

5. How can I be involved in planning the transition and preparing my child for the transition?

Just as in the earlier transition from early intervention to preschool, your consent should be obtained for release of information. Eligibility for continued services should be assessed well in advance of the transition to allow time to plan for the child's needs. Likewise, you should have the option of visiting programs, meeting with staff and sharing information about your child. Procedures should be developed to prepare your child for the change in programs, including ways to help your child adjust to and function well in the new program. The same seven steps recommended in planning the transition from early intervention services to preschool are recommended for planning the transition from preschool to kindergarten.

TRANSITIONS DUE TO FAMILY MOVES

Our society is very mobile and each year many families relocate to new neighborhoods, towns and even states. If you move during your child's first five years of life, how can you ensure that your child continues to receive appropriate services?

There is no requirement that programs develop formal transition plans when families move. However, typically your service provider will assist you in planning, if you ask. Just as during the transition at age three or five, you should request a meeting to discuss your child's records and to plan for a change in programs. Ask for a copy of the records, so that you may take them with you to your new home. If you are moving to a new state, you will need to find out what the eligibility requirements for services are. Your current provider may know; if not, most states have a 1-800 number for Child Find—a program to identify children who may be eligible for special education services. Call the State Department of Education in your new state and ask for the Child-Find number. The operator for the 1-800 number should be able to send you information about eligibility and whom to contact in your new town.

If possible, call the agency responsible for providing or coordinating early intervention or preschool services in your new town, before you move. Tell them when you are planning to move and ask them what information they would like in advance. You may be able to begin planning before the actual move. Your current program may be able to share information and also talk with your child's potential service provider. It's best to contact the new agency as soon as possible, as it may take some time to plan for and identify new services.

You should prepare your child for the separation from his current program and talk about his new program. Again, it may be helpful to visit potential programs once you have moved and to discuss with staff how the program can meet your child's needs. Once you have selected a program, plan to visit the new program with your child to introduce him to staff and classrooms. Be sure to exchange information about your child with the new staff and what you can do at home to support him in adjusting to the new program. As with any change, maintain communication with the new staff and expect the adjustment to take some time— for you and your child.

SUMMARY

During your child's first five years of life, you will change service providers several times. Changes in services can be a positive sign that your child is growing and developing. Changes also can be challenging, as you work to ensure that your child continues to receive the most appropriate services. You have the right to be involved in all decisions involved in the transition from one service program to another. This chapter has described some ways in which you may choose to be involved.

CHAPTER 9

Due Process

Patricia A. Edmister

In an ideal world, young children would not have disabilities which make early intervention and special education necessary. Unfortunately, that world does not exist for many families. Also, in a "somewhat ideal world", if a youngster was found to have a disability warranting intervention or special education, that service would be readily available and extremely comprehensive, providing everything parents and professionals believed would be beneficial to the child. Again, even that "somewhat ideal world" doesn't exist for many families. In those cases, parents may find themselves in disagreement with service providers over some aspect or aspects of their child's eligibility for services, or over what those services should consist of.

Fortunately, the federal law (described in Chapter 2) which authorizes early intervention and special education for infants and children with disabilities includes provisions which provide mechanisms for parents to seek "Due Process" proceedings by which to settle these disputes. This federal law is implemented on a state by state basis; thus, the way in which due process provisions are carried out will vary slightly from state to state. Some states, because of the newness of enactment of the full provisions of Part H (the infant and toddler provision) of the IDEA (Individuals with Disabilities Education Act), have not developed procedures for due process for infants and toddlers and their families, but that does not mean that you cannot seek resolution of your disagreements. If you need help in determining procedures, contact the lead agency in your state (for children under three) and the state education agency (for children over three) (see the appendix for identification of a contact person, or contact your Governor's office for the contact agency's name and number).

Why Parents Exercise Due Process Rights

There are many reasons parents may need to pursue their due process rights. Part H requires that participating states must serve infants from birth through age two who are "experiencing developmental delays" or "who have a diagnosed physical or mental condition which has a high probability of resulting in developmental delay". It also requires that each state develop a definition of "developmentally delayed infants and toddlers". A more difficult component of the act gives states discretion as to whether or not they will serve infants and toddlers "who are at **risk** of having substantial developmental delays if early intervention services are not provided". Many of the disputes leading to requests for due process hearings revolve around the following issues:

1. Disputes between parents and service providers regarding:

- Is the child truly experiencing developmental delays?

- Is the child only at risk for delays and, by a particular state's definition, thereby ineligible?

- What exactly should that program consist of? (If both parents and service providers agree that the child is eligible for some service)

2. Disagreement Over Evaluation and Assessment

Some disputes occur quite early in the identification process itself. To answer the first question, **"Is the child truly delayed?"** assessment and diagnosis is the first step. As was discussed in Chapter 5, assessment and diagnosis of young children are difficult due to the limited number of assessment instruments appropriate for children in this age bracket, the complexities and irregularities in early childhood development, a lack of reliable information concerning the relationship between various social, biological and medical factors which contribute to disabilities in early childhood, and the lack of agreement among professionals about what constitutes "normal" levels of performance in infants and toddlers.

A recent study by the Carolina Policy Studies Program found that while most states' definitions of what constituted a developmental delay were very similar to the wording of Part H, the definitions changed considerably once eligibility criteria were examined. In fact, the researchers found very little agreement from state to state regarding specific criteria being used.

What happens, then, is that a child may be eligible for services under the guidelines in one state, and yet be ineligible for services in another. For example, one state may determine that a child is eligible if he is delayed by 25% in one area whereas another state may require a delay of 50%. Still another may require a delay of 25% in two or more areas. Obviously, this can result in rather significant differences of opinion as to what in fact should constitute a developmental delay, and thus, eligibility for services between parents and service providers who are trying to follow the state guidelines.

Since, as stated above, it is so difficult to measure a young child's performance levels on many of the tests used, the results of such assessment may be suspect in terms of accuracy. Another problem can arise when a child moves from infant/toddler to preschool services. Since there are somewhat different eligibility requirements under the sections of the law which cover these two age groups, some children who were eligible for services as infants may not be eligible as preschoolers. Thus, parents whose child comes close to meeting eligibility standards but doesn't quite qualify, may object to the finding of ineligibility.

PROVISION OF SERVICES FOR AN ELIGIBLE INFANT, TODDLER, OR PRESCHOOLER.

Even though evaluation and assessment may have shown that a child meets the state's criteria for eligibility, there may then be disagreement among professionals over what **are** appropriate services to provide to the youngster and his or her family to meet the identified needs.

It is this disagreement among professionals that often confuses and frustrates parents who have been told by one set of knowledgeable professionals that their child needs one level of service, yet are then confronted by another set of professionals who say that this child needs a different level of service. In most, although not all cases, the level suggested by the service providers is less than that recommended by the other health and educational professionals; thus, there is disagreement.

Such disagreements usually focus on issues such as:

1. How many days per week will the child receive service?

2. Where will the service be provided? Center/Site-based or home-based?

3. Who will be providing the services? What are their qualifications?

4.   What related services will be provided and how frequently?

When to Exercise Your Due Process Rights

The decision to exercise one's due process rights is often an agonizing one. Many parents are quite concerned that by doing so, they may in some way jeopardize their child's right to receive services. This should never be the case. The right to due process was designed to allow for appropriate complaint resolution. Just as the child has the right to remain in his program receiving the services which are **not** in dispute, so too, do parents have the right to timely, appropriate complaint resolution. One less adversarial option available in many states is to pursue mediation instead of a due process hearing. This may turn out to be a step prior to initiation of the due process hearing option (which is usually a fairly formal route to pursue), or may in fact result in dispute resolution without the more difficult, time consuming Due Process Hearing.

What is Mediation?

While the process of mediation varies from jurisdiction to jurisdiction, typically mediation is a "voluntary form of complaint resolution which protects the child's interests while helping parents and service providers reach a mutually agreeable decision" (Maryland Infants and Toddler's Program brochure entitled: "Mediation in the Early Intervention System"). This process is much less formal than a due process hearing, but can be equally effective in obtaining results. Trained mediators are used to encourage and facilitate discussion, make suggestions regarding areas of dispute, and generally to help maintain a collaborative relationship to assist the parties in coming to a mutually satisfactory conclusion.

Mediation typically takes less time than a hearing and is much less expensive for the various parties concerned, especially if attorneys become involved. Attorney fees are not reimbursed to parents pursuing due process hearings under Part H (birth to three). In contrast, those fees are reimbursed to the prevailing party under Part B, for children of ages three to 21). In most states offering mediation, it can be terminated by either party if there is dissatisfaction with the process or the progress. If agreement is not reached, the parties are advised by the mediator of the next step in the complaint resolution process - a due process hearing.

The Due Process Hearing

A due process hearing can be a very emotionally draining experience, both as one prepares for it, and as one participates in it. If you prepare carefully for it in terms of collecting information about your child, getting appropriate expert witnesses to assist you in interpreting assessment information and/performance information, you can minimize the negative impact it might have on you and your family members.

Parents have the right to request a hearing when there is a dispute over any of the aforementioned areas. The actual process for filing a request varies from state to state and local jurisdictions in terms of what applications to file and to whom they should be sent. Parents should contact their local lead agency if the child is under three, or the state educational agency for information if the child is over three, for information on how to file. At that time, the parents should also be informed by the lead agency or the public school system (or should ask) of all the procedural safeguards available to them, including information on how to proceed and in what time frame the other party must respond, and when/where the due process hearings take place.

Beginning the Process

You will have to submit your request in writing, to the local lead agency or to a body so empowered by the state (Part H, birth through age two) or to the school system (Part B, three to 21). This is usually done by completing a form provided by the agency. It is important to be mindful of timelines which you should observe and which the other party must observe.

Once the process is initiated, the timeline begins. A hearing date is scheduled and an impartial hearing officer is selected from a list maintained by the agency or state. *Impartial* means that the hearing officer may not be an employee of the agency involved or have any conflict of interest in serving in this role that might jeopardize his or her objectivity. In some states, these hearing officers are former judges; in others they are individuals with specialized training and expertise in special education. In some jurisdictions, legal counsel may be hired by the lead agency or school system to assist the hearing officers by providing specialized information regarding special education legislation and case law. Such counsel is to remain neutral, merely assisting the hearing officers in understanding the law.

Either party in the dispute may choose to be represented by an attorney and has the right to call witnesses. Legal representation does add to the cost of the proceedings and, under part H (birth through two), is **not** reimbursable to parents if they prevail, unlike provisions of Part B (three to 21) which reimburse parents for costs incurred if they prevail in the dispute. Nevertheless, in complex cases, participation of an attorney experienced in special education due process procedures may be beneficial to your family during both the preparation phase and during the actual hearing. In some locales, there are parent or child advocates who are also well acquainted with special education law. They too can be extremely helpful to a family during this process.

Often, especially in more rural locales, it is difficult to find expert witnesses, parent advocates, and/or special education attorneys. One possible source is to contact the service delivery provider that parents are hoping will provide services to the child in the future and determine if personnel from that program might serve as witnesses. In addition, the program's administrator usually has information regarding parent advocates and/or attorneys with whom they have had contact in previous disputes. Parents might also consult with other parents of children in various programs for advice regarding witnesses, etc. or contact local parent groups, such as the Association for Retarded Citizens or parents of Down Syndrome children for advice.

Preparing for the Hearing

In many ways, the preparation phase of the due process hearing is the most important because the information you accumulate will form the basis upon which the hearing officer will make his or her decision. This information will consist of assessments, physician's reports, pupil progress reports (if child is currently enrolled in a program) and any other documents you plan to make available. It will also include decisions on your part regarding the use of expert witnesses and the content of their testimony.

Once again, it is important to be mindful of timelines and begin your preparation in a timely fashion, for things can get lost in the mail, you may have difficulty contacting your experts, etc.

The Role of the Case Presenter

Parents must decide who will present their position to the hearing officer. This person is responsible, in most cases, for both the preparation and presentation of information. This may be a parent, an advocate representing the family, or an attorney. This person's responsibilities include: becoming familiar with all aspects of the case and the issues which are being challenged; choosing appropriate documents; determining whether or not expert witnesses will be called and, if so, preparing them for testifying; and preparing for and conducting any prehearing meetings of the individuals involved in the case where strategies may be determined and presentation order will be decided upon.

Choosing Documents

Documentation to support your point of view in the case is extremely important, for it gives the hearing officer a frame of reference and a historical perspective about your child. The documentation should include information about the child's disabilities, any educational assessments or interventions that have been offered, and what have been the areas of disagreement between the two parties in the case. Materials should be arranged in chronological order and include information documenting the child's service history, the child's disability (reports such as educational assessments, medical reports, reports of other evaluators such as speech pathologists or occupational therapists, etc.) and information regarding the concerns, priorities, and resources of the family (under Part H; birth through two).

The service delivery system will also prepare documents and you are entitled to copies of all of those materials by requesting them from the service delivery provider. In addition, the service provider typically will provide a description of the program or services being proposed by them to meet the child's needs.

You, however, may have descriptions of other services or programs you and your witnesses feel are more appropriate to meet your child's needs. Information about those programs should be included, or you may wish to have a witness called to speak to those program's services relative to your child's needs.

Choosing Witnesses

The selection of witnesses is a critical piece of the hearing preparation process. Their ability to testify clearly and concisely regarding your child's needs, and their ability to respond professionally under cross-examination can affect the outcome. Everyone needs to be aware that nervousness, anxiety, defensiveness, outright fear and conflict of interest concerns can all affect your witness's testimony. In addition, having expert witnesses available can be a costly proposition so choose carefully.

Know the Facts of the Case

It is very important that you, your witnesses, and your attorney/case presenter (if not yourself) know the facts of the case. Everyone should have reviewed all documents in your child's record and any written information the service provider plans to submit (which should be requested at the time of filing for a due process hearing). If you are planning to have expert witnesses testify about documents they have prepared or tests they have given to the child, they need to be prepared to answer technical questions about the reliability and validity of the instruments used and why that was the test of choice.

If you are proposing an alternative placement for the child, you should have someone available to discuss why that placement is necessary and what it can provide that the other one can't. This may be specific instructional techniques or special related services.

The Prehearing Briefing

Once all pertinent documents are collected and witnesses selected, a prehearing briefing should be held. This is an opportunity for everyone to prepare their testimony for the hearing. It should be held enough in advance of the hearing to allow for additional preparation or document selection if needed. Witnesses must have an opportunity for complete discussion of the issues of the case. Each person should be given a chance to express his or her opinions and testimony should then be discussed.

The order of witnesses must be considered. The lead witness is quite important, for this person often sets the tone of the case, so select someone who is comfortable with the hearing process. Usually the first witness presents a chronology of the child's past education and progress, if the child has been receiving service. The next witnesses usually address the child's disability and provide evaluation data to support that identification. The last witnesses are usually service providers who will discuss what services are needed.

To prepare your witnesses for testifying, develop a series of questions for them designed to help them present their professional qualifications and to give them opportunities to offer clear statements regarding their involvement in this case. Witnesses must also be prepared to handle cross-examination by representatives of the other side. During the briefing, possible questions should be considered and role-playing should be done to help witnesses be familiar with the process and their feelings. Witness preparation is a critical component of the prehearing briefing, for this is the time to allay fears and anxieties.

For many first time witnesses, there is tremendous anxiety upon realizing that they are about to present their professional credentials for scrutiny and possible criticism, and that they must not appear defensive. Some witnesses are actually afraid of being asked questions. For these individuals, you need to be supportive and caring. In extreme cases, you may need to consider finding another witness who is more comfortable with the process. With all witnesses, role playing simulations in front of colleagues until the person feels comfortable can help build self confidence in the witness.

THE HEARING

Pre-hearing Preparation

The night before the hearing,

1. read all the documents
2. outline your responses
3. list relevant facts upon which you will be testifying
4. get a good night's sleep

General Instructions for Testifying

1. Answer all questions clearly and concisely.
2. Present information in a straightforward, professional manner, citing support documents when relevant.
3. Stay within the context of the question asked.

4. Take your time in preparing to answer the question to get organized.

(From: *Preparing for Special Education Hearing: A Practical Guide to Lessening the Trauma of Due Process Hearings* by Richard E. Ekstrand, Patricia Edmister, and Jane Riggin, published by the Council for Exceptional Children, 1989)

Demeanor during the Hearing

The demeanor of witnesses can contribute to its effective resolution, especially if the witnesses do not seem to take it seriously. Remind your witnesses that this is a somewhat formal process and that they should act accordingly, maintaining their professionalism and composure.

Direct and Cross Examination

Witnesses should be well prepared from the pre-hearing briefing for what will be their testimony. They may refer to notes and documents. During cross examination, witnesses should respond as follows: (From Ekstrand, Edmister and Riggin, 1989):

1. Give honest, succinct and sufficient answers to questions without volunteering irrelevant information. Listen carefully to the question and ask for clarification if needed.

2. Defer to another witness if necessary and appropriate.

3. Take time to reflect before answering.

4. Do not be defensive.

5. Say "I don't know" if that is the case, and then leave it at that.

6. Do not respond to silence. If the witness responds unnecessarily during a time gap, the responses will sometimes elicit additional questions that can prove troublesome.

7. Ask clarifying questions if you are unclear about the question being asked or if it has multiple parts.

Post-Hearing Behavior

One of the most difficult aspects of the hearing process for parents and providers is the emotional tension felt between them both during the hearing itself, and even more, following completion of the hearing — before and after the decision has been announced. A primary goal of both parties should be, for the sake of the child and in the interest of future working relationships, to keep negative feelings towards each other to a minimum. This can be very difficult, for often statements are made by witnesses on each side that question the motives or competencies of those involved. The feelings these statements generate may contribute to difficulty in establishing or maintaining a positive, beneficial coopera-tive relationship. It is critical, however, that all parties make a strong effort to create a good working relationship for the benefit of the child.

While you are waiting for the outcome of the hearing, your child's program should continue without interruption (if he is currently in a placement). During this time, it is most important that the two parties strive to work together to minimize as much as possible any adverse effects on the child. Once the hearing results are announced, regardless of the findings, service providers should maintain their professionalism and parents should work with the appropriate personnel to implement the child's determined program. All must work towards putting nega-tive feelings behind them with the goal of providing an appropriate program from which your child can benefit.

If the relationship remains strained despite efforts to improve it, it may be helpful to bring in a program administrator or a counselor to facilitate improving interactions.

Next Steps

Once the hearing results are returned, the determined action is to take place as quickly as possible. If you disagree with the decisions, you do have the right to then pursue an appeal. In most states appeals are made to a higher educational hearing board. If you disagree with the results of that appeal, you have the right to pursue civil court action.

CONCLUSION

Hearings are a critical component of your right to due process, yet they can be very emotional, draining activities. The goal is to attain an appropriate educational program for your child. Although it may take time and lots of preparation to do that, if you prevail the outcome makes it worthwhile.

CHAPTER 10

Opening Many, Many Doors: Parent-to-Parent Support

Patricia McGill Smith

Parents and families go through a crisis when their child is identified as having a disability. I would like to share with you some of my personal experiences in this field. The experiences come from being the parent of a daughter with disabilities and having worked in a variety of parent support programs at all levels. My experience started with the Pilot Parent Program in Omaha, Nebraska and progressed to Deputy Assistant Secretary of the Office of Special Education and Rehabilitative Services of the U.S. Department of Education. My current position as Executive Director of the National Parent Network on Disabilities (NPND) has returned me to that aspect of supporting parents and families which I consider the most personally rewarding.

As a result of the help Jane, my family and I, have received, we have had the privilege to pass through many doors. This chapter represents an opportunity to present personal reflections and programmatic information to help other parents of children with disabilities convert what may appear to them as a bureaucratic barrier into a series of open doors and supportive experiences.

To begin, I would like to share portions of an article I wrote entitled *"You are Not Alone"*, a Bulletin for Parents of Children with Disabilities. This paper was written when I left Omaha, Nebraska, my home, to move to Washington D.C. It was a compilation of thoughts distilled during the first 10 years of my career helping parents of children with disabilities. My intention was to share my experience, strength and hope to help other parents.

"When parents learn about any difficulty or problem in their child's development, this information comes as a tremendous blow......I was devastated - and so confused.... I recall little else about those first days other than the heartbreak. Another parent described this event as a 'black sack' being pulled down over her head, blocking her ability to hear, see and think in normal ways. Another parent described the trauma as 'having a knife stuck' in her heart. Perhaps these descriptions seem a bit dramatic, yet it has been my experience that they may not sufficiently describe the many emotions that flood parents' minds and hearts when they receive any bad news about their child."

"The feeling of isolation at the time of diagnosis is almost a universal feeling among parents.....You can diminish these feelings by recognizing that they have been experienced by many, many others, that understanding and constructive help are available to you and your child, and you are not alone."

"This person is your child, first and foremost. Granted, your child's development may be different from that of other children, but this does not make your child less valuable, less human, less important, or less in need of your love and parenting. Love and enjoy your child. The child comes first; the disabling condition is second. If you can relax and take positive steps...one at a time, you will do the best you can, your child will benefit, and you can look forward to the future with hope."

MY JANE

I would like to begin my sharing by telling you my personal experiences with my seventh child, Jane (now twenty-two years old). Jane's birth was what I consider to be a perfect, unmedicated, spontaneous birth. All was well. However, within the first two months, I noticed differences. By six months, I was alarmed. I questioned the doctor: "Is she deaf? Is she blind? Are her legs working? Why doesn't she roll over or sit?" I also asked many other questions. He and the other doctors I consulted kept telling me Jane was within the normal range of development. They told me to come back when Jane reached age one. I took Jane to the doctor on her first birthday, looking again for a diagnosis. Once more I was put off.

By the time Jane reached her first birthday, I had worn the doctor out with questions about her development. My mother's heart knew something different. I desperately wanted to believe the doctor's assessment of her development, "She's functioning within her age range, she is experiencing some developmental delays." But I really didn't believe him.

The first year of her life was a long and lonely one for me. I was drawing farther and farther away from people. I didn't want to talk about Jane. It got to the point I really couldn't talk to anyone. My children were too young to understand or to be burdened with my fears. My husband always relied on "what the doctor said".

My best friend also had a daughter named Jane. She was 2 months older than my Jane. It was very hard to see or hear about the accomplishments of the other Jane. When my friend's daughter was a year old she was off, running all over and talking up a storm. The only way my Jane could get around was to roll like a little log. She was very proficient at it, but then she learned how to commando crawl. You know, flat on your tummy, pulling her body along with her elbows and arms. Jane got really good at it too.

When Jane was 8 months old, I had to leave her with my best friend and her daughter Jane. When I returned, a day later, my best friend was crying. She had cried a lot that day. She told me, "There is something the matter with your Jane. She needs help."

Armed with the observation and concern of my best friend, I attacked the doctor with more questions. The doctor promised me he would give me answers when Jane turned one. So I took Jane to the doctor on her first birthday for his answers. He had no answers. I was very angry. That was the day I decided to do something to help me figure out what was wrong with Jane.

I went to the telephone book and looked up "Pediatricians". I remember reading the list, recognizing many of the names. I saw the name of the one I had taken Jane to when she was seven months old...he was no help. One name stood out. People called him the "pediatrician's pediatrician". I called for an appointment. I had to wait 2 very long months.

On a very hot afternoon, late in July, I went with Jane to see this new doctor. As I look back now, this would be the first of many, many doors she and I would go through, together.

The doctor was a tall man. We stood next to each other as he examined Jane on the table. I stood close to Jane because she was always unhappy in new places and with new people. After a few minutes, the doctor turned and looked me right in the face and said, "It's simple, mother. This child is retarded." As he spoke, I can remember the hot tears streaming down my face. He kept talking about how he thought, "She could learn, she could stay at home, and all those brother and sisters would be a terrific asset." When I kept questioning him about when and what were we to do, he responded, "Take her home and keep her comfortable. When she is three or four years old, see if you can find a preschool for her."

I can't remember much else about that day, except for the awful shock of the news. I do recall driving home with Jane beside me. I cried all the way home. I cried all day and all night. I don't remember telling anyone about her "problem"....I know I did tell her dad, but the details I can't remember.

The next morning was my niece's wedding. It was a huge wedding and all of the family was to go to this wonderful party. My mother always taught us, "When a problem arises and you don't know what to do, then do whatever it was that you were going to do anyway." Practicing this habit seems to produce some normalcy and consistency when life becomes hectic. This was good advice and that's what we did. Jane went to the sitter. The rest of us went to the wedding.

That day was a blurred memory. People kept patting me on the shoulder and no one wanted to look into my eyes. It was a strange feeling to be carrying such a sadness and loss at a time of joy and celebration. We tried to carry it off as best we could. I remember a few words, "It's good she doesn't look retarded." That stung. There were many concerns about what this problem child would cost. In the mid afternoon, my brother asked me to talk to friends we knew during childhood, Joe and Ginny Friend. They had information that might help us with Jane. Were Jane's Daddy and I willing to talk to them? YES!

That conversation with the Friends is forever as burned into my memory as was the doctor's diagnosis the day before. The Friends explained they had an 8-year-old son named Matthew who had mental retardation and unfortunately, because he was so hard to manage, they placed him at the Beatrice State Developmental Center in Beatrice, Nebraska.

Joe Friend asked me all about the diagnosis and what Jane could do. When I said the doctor thought she could learn, he said, "Good, that's great." When I said the doctor thought she could live at home and our large family was a tremendous blessing, he responded, "That's wonderful. What a good prognosis. Yes, your family will be of help. There are many others who will help you. There are programs and support services. You aren't alone in this. There is help." And his final remark, "You may bless the day she was born and be grateful she is your daughter and a part of your family." I could hardly believe my ears. He was talking about hope and help and services and positive things. I didn't bless her birth that day...but I have always thanked God for the gift of the Friends. This couple produced a ray of sunshine, a message of hope for the future.

I ran on automatic for days, doing the things I could do without much thought. Everything was a blur. I don't remember much, only lots of tears. Everyone who tried to "help" could only tell me stories of someone they knew who had someone in their family who had mental retardation. That did not help.

A few days later, Fran Porter called me. She also was a parent of a child with mental retardation. She was positive and encouraging, like Joe and Ginny Friend. In both meetings, I was encouraged to get help for Jane, as soon as possible. I kept calling the doctor about a referral for help. He stuck to his original advice, "Wait two or three years and then take her to a preschool. Keep her comfortable and love her." This conflict in advice made me more depressed. I couldn't call my family doctor because I walked away from his care to get the diagnosis from the new doctor. More depression.

It took six weeks for me to make a decision. Actually, the first opportunity to act on my decision came when two of the older children were having tubes put in their ears at a hospital directly across the street from the center Fran Porter had recommended. As soon as they were wheeled off to surgery, I made a beeline for the front door of the Meyer Children's Rehabilitation Institute (MCRI) at the University of Nebraska Medical Center. Unannounced and unreferred (except by a parent) I approached the reception desk and announced, "I've been told you help children. I have a child "they" say has mental retardation. Can you help me?"

I, we, Jane and I....our whole family has been receiving help ever since. During the following months Jane was enrolled in a research program at MCRI. During those early months and years, I became an integral part of Jane's support team. With very skillful teachers and support I began to accept Jane Smith, and to rethink my dreams and expectations. At first, I was quite alone in my quest to help Jane. The therapists and teachers worked individually with us. Eventually, the seeds of acceptance of Jane began to spread through our family and friends. Acceptance of her allowed her dad, brothers and sisters to join as a part of the support team to help Jane. Often these were long and lonely days that turned to happier, productive, engaging times where each family member learned to play and feel a sense of pride and joy at Jane's accomplishments. During the time spent at MCRI, I started to meet other families. We "coffeed" together and formed circles of friendship around our children and their siblings. We talked...WE TALKED A LOT!

At the age of two, Jane started crawling on her hands and knees like crazy, but of course the other Jane had been walking and running for a year.

The way I finally got Jane to start walking was to stand her up against a wall and make her reach out for Cheerios to take one step and then another. Whether this was right or wrong in a "professional's" mind, Jane finally walked. I bribed her with Cheerios, but she walked! The stark contrast between my Jane and my best friend's Jane then and even now, leaves a small hurt deep inside, but I love them both.

When Jane was four, our family was in the middle of a crisis. The children's father was hospitalized for a long stay. The term of his employment was very unstable. My only option was to find a job.

There was an advertisement in a flyer from the Association for Retarded Citizens (ARC) requesting a coordinator for the Pilot Parent Program for the Greater Omaha Association for Retarded Citizens. I knew Pilot Parents helped parents, but I had never been officially involved in their services. Thinking this was a part-time, not-too-demanding job, I decided to apply. (Little did I know.) There were three requirements: 1) college degree or some college training; 2) membership in the Pilot Parents, and 3) being the parent of a child with a disability. I missed the first two, but made the third one. When I called, the person on the other end of the phone said the first two qualifications were negotiable but not the third. You had to be a parent of a child with a disability to get the job.

In October, I went to work for Pilot Parents. From the day I started, I've remembered the blessed help of Joe and Ginny Friend and Fran Porter to get me/us through the early days after Jane's diagnosis. Is it any surprise that in 1971 when I was helped, Joe Friend was the President of the Greater Omaha Association for Retarded Citizens (GOARC) and Fran Porter along with Shirley Dean and Dr. Wolf Wolfensburger were developing and implementing the first Pilot Parents. When the Friends helped me, they were operating as Pilot Parents before the official program began.

THE IDEA

The Pilot Parent Program is the original concept which has been the model for most of the parent-helping-parent programs across the country and around the world. Fran Porter's idea was that was when parents find out they have a child with a disability, they should not be alone in their search for help. She believed the information she learned through personal experience with her child would be valuable for other parents. Shirley Dean and Dr. Wolfensburger, both professionals, agreed. (Shirley Dean wanted to organize the emotional support and role modeling for parents comparable to the support provided by professionals.) Dr. Wolfensburger wanted to organize a total community support system for parents and family members. The three original concepts were blended to create Pilot Parents.

As with many people helping people situations, the Parent-to-Parent Program has been formalized for some time. Since my experience in the early 70's, literally hundreds of such organizations have sprung up around the world.

THE PHILOSOPHY OF THE PILOT PARENT PROGRAM

The Pilot Parent Program is based on the philosophy that parents of children with developmental disabilities who are experiencing crisis can be helped by other parents who have made an exemplary adjustment to their own child. These "veteran" parents often have the capacity and willingness to help others by sharing their experiences. These parents share, too, their belief every child is a valuable and developing person, who is entitled to develop to his fullest potential. We also believe the child is entitled to receive services in a setting which is least restrictive based on his or her individual needs. Further, Pilot Parents believe in sharing their knowledge with new parents so no child will be institutionalized due to lack of awareness of services in the community. We also believe parents participating as pilot parents will produce a metamorphosis of attitudes, values, capabilities, concerns, and involvement creating a common bond which draws parents, their families and the community closer to one another.

The Need for Support

Parents who have just received the news their child has a disability are often traumatized for a period of time. They feel alone, helpless and completely uninformed. They need someone to talk to who really understands what they're going through. Historically, the parent-to-parent movement has demonstrated that talking to a parent of a child with a similar disability provides a level of support unlike that attained by talking to almost anyone else. Hence, the first priority of a parent-to-parent support program is the linking of parents of children with similar disabilities to each other. The key to effective support is to understand that support is a delicately balanced service which mixes emotional stability with factual resource information. Effective support is empowering. It provides the *new parent* with the understanding there is hope. It provides information, opinions and attitudes with which the *new parent* can make more informed judgments and take action on behalf of their child. The business of providing effective support is a tricky one. Hence, the need for the comprehensive training and support of the volunteer parents.

ESTABLISHING PARENT-TO-PARENT SUPPORT GROUPS

What You Need to Know

The following steps summarize the action parents can take to learn how to establish parent to parent support organizations and program features which have proven critical to the success of such programs.

Contact the Parent Training and Information Center in Your State

Each state and some U.S. territories have a Parent Training and Information Center. These centers exist for the express purpose of providing formalized information about special education, training and support to parents of children with disabilities. They will be able to identify existing Parent to Parent Programs in your state or provide you with information on how to start one. If you do not know how to locate or contact the Parent Training and Information Center in your state, contact your State Department of Education, Special Education Division or contact the National Parent Network on Disabilities. The address and telephone numbers of these resources are provided in the Appendix of this book. In your state, there may be more than one community with an active Parent-to-Parent Program. Contact the one closest to you and learn about their activities.

If there is no program in your area and you want to create one, keep in mind the following components.

Recruiting and Training Volunteer Parents

In order to assure that parents offer support and empowerment to the *new parents*, it is important to put in place an effective training program. Such training should accomplish four goals:

1) Assure that volunteer parents who are linked to *new parents* know how to handle emotionally charged situations.

2) Assure that parents know about and have access to all resources and services which are available to assist *new parents*. (Department of Social Services, Special Education Law, Early Childhood Education Programs, Respite Care, etc.).

3) Train volunteer parents in a variety of disabilities, or at least be able to provide them with information about the specific disabilities. Volunteers should also know the characteristics of the service system responding to the *new parent's* child's particular disability, if different from the more generalized service system. It is wise to use parent trainers who have had interaction with the specific service systems so they can describe how they negotiated the system for their family member.

4) Provide an opportunity for parents who are not yet ready or comfortable providing direct support to identify other ways they can participate in the program.

Careful Screening

It is important that parents offering support to *new parents* clearly demonstrate she/he has already been where the *new parent* is headed. It is also important they have made it successfully through the program and are ready to work with a family.

Careful Matching

It is important that parents needing support be carefully matched with parents of children with the same or similar disability, and if possible, within the same socio-economic, ethnic or language background.

Empowerment

The *new parent* should direct the support services they receive. While *new parents* may at first welcome any help they can get, they will soon identify and communicate their specific needs. To be effective, it is necessary for the parent offering support to recognize and acknowledge the direction of the *new parent*. By doing so, the *new parent* is empowered through the recognition of the experienced parent that they are able to take over.

The above characteristics are only key characteristics that effective parent to parent programs possess. They have been used over and over and elaborated on for years to develop programs around the world.

HOW TO GET STARTED

To ensure a program for parent-to-parent support not only exists but flourishes and is maintained the following steps should be taken:

• *Establish a Network*
Identify other parents and/or support organizations who may wish to participate in the creation of a parent-to-parent support program. In establishing a parent-to-parent support group it is essential all interested parties in the community have an opportunity to participate in its creation. Be sure to involve professionals who will recognize the benefits of a parent-to-parent program and can lend valuable expertise as consultants and/or make resources available to the program. By using a thorough networking base, word of your intentions will reach a wider audience. You may find support from places you never thought to look. The use of a network will hopefully prevent you from missing potential members. Include as many key groups as possible to ensure a very broad base of resource support for the program.

Remember, parents and family members of children with disabilities are everywhere. Use organizational newsletters, put an article in the local newspaper, PTA groups, school district newsletters to let everyone know what is going to happen and invite them to participate.

• *Find a sponsor*
In order to give the program a stable base, it may be necessary to attach it to an existing organization, or if necessary, create a new organization.

While there are pros and cons to forming a new organization rather than connecting with an existing one, probably the better course is to start the program with a friendly sponsor organization. At a later date, spin the parent-to-parent program off into its own free standing structure. Connecting with an existing organization will help you set up the business systems you will need to attract and account for the resources you will use to provide support. It is important, of course, to pick the sponsoring organization carefully. It is preferable the sponsor have a non-profit, 501(c)3 status.

• *Establish an operational structure*

The organizational structure will vary depending on the needs of the membership and community and should be carefully thought out to best address the number and variety of needs identified in the community. Contact existing Parent to Parent groups in and out of your state, with a similar community size or sponsoring organization. There are good programs out there who are more than happy to share information. Use the resources of the Parent Training and Information Center in your state to contact other programs and help you build the structure. Also, use the National Center On Parent Directed Family Resource Centers in San Jose, California and/or the National Parent Network on Disabilities for technical assistance.

• *Develop a Budget and Support Staff*

While parents of children with disabilities should be involved in all of the organizational planning, they do not have time to oversee the day to day activities of a project like this. The sponsoring organization can help you establish a budget. They may also be able to provide a staff person who can coordinate the program. The coordinator can work directly with the parent volunteers, oversee the day to day work, help set up the training schedule for the volunteer parents, assist in the matching of volunteer parents to *new parents*, and help identify possible funding sources to support the program. Parents can assist the staff person. Perhaps the staff person could be a parent who has time available or is looking for a part-time job.

The program need not be a high cost program. At a minimum, it could support volunteers by paying mileage expenses, postage and printing. On the other hand, you may want to develop a very sophisticated organization with a full support staff. It does require a high degree of commitment and resources so all are involved to support the program. Make sure the volunteer duties are spread around so individual parents don't "burn out". As you experience success and the demand for experienced parents grows, it will be necessary to identify funding sources to assure activities such as recruiting and matching occur. You will want to be sure your training meets the need of volunteers both in content, quantity and quality. Finally, it is important that requests from *new parents* receive a prompt response and the daily activities required to support the program are assured.

Your local program should be designed to fit the needs of your community. But if the basic characteristics and steps are followed, the rest will fall into place.

RESULTS OF THE PARENT-TO-PARENT MOVEMENT

The parent-to-parent model has been a springboard for the development of many parent/professional partnerships. The Parent Information and Training Centers and 350 Parent Helping Parent Programs located in every state and several territories, and the National Parent Network on Disabilities have incorporated many of these concepts. There has been an effort to include families from many cultures so the program is supportive to all families. Technology has allowed us to make available all the information and materials to families in their native language. In some of the parent centers there is specific training and trainers for different cultures.

Parents have become more involved in school community programs as well as the day-to-day needs of their children. They are now becoming involved in the governmental process of program development for persons with disabilities. Parents have found they do have a voice to influence and bring about change. Parents and families have now reached into all the service agencies. They are beginning to have representation on local, state and federal committees, task forces, review teams, and participate in grant and research development.

As indicated throughout this book, current laws have parents heavily involved from the very beginning. The development of the Individual Family Service Plan (IFSP) involves the family from the beginning of the development of the educational plan for their child.

The impact on the child whose parents have been involved from the beginning is much stronger. Parents have a more normal life cycle with the child and they have higher expectations for the child. Parents are becoming more sophisticated and can view their child more objectively. They can look to the future with more joy, and less stress and disappointment.

Future: More To Do

There is still more work to be done to help parents across the country. There needs to be national unity. Parents from all over come together every two years to celebrate themselves at the National Parent to Parent Conference. It should happen every year, not only nationally, but in each state. Parents need the time to celebrate, to share, to meet others, and to network. There needs to be definitive research on the outcome of parent-to-parent programs. What is happening to the families currently in programs? What has happened with the children, their school programs, their community involvement, their transition to adult life? Each state needs a statewide coalition of parent groups. Parents in states need to network, communicate and share. There needs to be parent-driven impact into the government on issues which affect persons with disabilities.

There is still a lot of work to do, but look how far we have come in twenty-two years. Think what it will be like in another twenty-two.

CHAPTER 11

Conclusion

By now it should be clear that as parents, you may have many rights within the early intervention program. In addition, there are many strategies you can use to take advantage of these rights and to make certain your child receives all the services to which he or she is entitled. As an informed parent you can be your child's most powerful advocate.

This book provides you with basic information in several key areas.

1. We have provided you with basic information about the laws relevant to young children with disabilities. The way each state implements services for young children varies. You should use the information about the federal laws in combination with information about the specific policies used in *your* state to provide services to your child.

2. We have reviewed the importance of becoming a keen observer of your child, both in the areas in which he or she is strong and those in which there are special needs. It will help to record these in as much detail as you can so you can remember them. You will want the evidence of your child's progress to assure that the program being developed or implemented is appropriate and challenging for your child. Children on sporadic hospital or clinic visits to a place that is strange, foreign and forbidding will often not display their finest accomplishments—perhaps not even in a preschool. Any delays also need attention. Again, your information from the home or your child's preschool or nursery may or may not reflect your perceptions. If you feel your judgments about your child's needs do not agree with the judgments of the professionals planning your child's program, your detailed observations of your child's behaviors will serve to support the position you see as critical to your child's progress.

   So, it is important:

   a. to observe and record your child's behavior carefully and regularly, especially instances of the behaviors you feel are especially important.

b. to integrate the information you have about your child and your family—in an ongoing fashion—so you can look backward and support statements of progress or continuing lack of progress in particular developmental areas.

This includes information about your child's likes and dislikes, your family's priorities and about your child's physical, developmental and emotional status.

c. to keep careful records that you can easily access and present. This is a major element in the informed discussions you can have with the service providers. It helps to keep records of contacts with the various professionals and the matters you discussed, their statements about you, your child and your family, and your thoughts about your reactions to those discussions. This will enable you to more dispassionately discuss these matters at the appropriate forums—your child's program planning meeting, discussions with the various professionals at your scheduled or unscheduled visits.

d. to realize that you don't need to wait for the scheduled visits with the staff working with your child or your family to occur. If you are concerned about aspects of your child's progress—or lack of progress—feel free to call for an appointment to talk about your concern— sooner rather than later.

3. The book has also provided you with information about what happens, and what you can expect to occur as your child moves into the service system. For example, most families are in contact with more than one service provider, must attend Individual Educational Plan (IEP) or Indivdual Family Service Plan (IFSP) meetings, and must face the periodic transition from the early childhood program to preschool and, then, school programs. It is much easier to be prepared when you are expecting these events and know something of what occurs at each point.

Finally, the book was intended to share strategies we have found useful. These include strategies for managing the piles of information and reports you will accumulate as you move though the process, strategies for handling yourself at IEP and IFSP meetings, and ways of getting support for yourself.

It is our hope you find the information in this book useful as you make your way through the service system. By developing an understanding of this system when your child is young, you are taking the first steps toward becoming an advocate for your child. It is important to realize that you serve a critical role in ensuring that this early intervention system the preschool system which follws, and the school system for the succeeding 17 years receives your input. Your active involvement will help ensure that the system is appropriate for *your* child and your family.

In short, as you enter the early intervention system you are embarking on a lengthy involvement on behalf of your child that only you—as parents—can engage in. Your involvement is important so that you can make sure this is done with an understanding of the needs of the entire family.

Politics, personalities and finances strongly influence actual outcomes. Individual providers often do not speak for or control the systems they operate in. Parents, standing outside the system, can help ensure these system factors do not derail their child's optimal course. Parents have a unique role to play and no one except your agents—people you may designate—can substitute for you. You *can* influence this process and help maximize your child's opportunities in the educational system. It will be an interesting journey for you—if often frustrating.

References

Anderson, W., Chitwood, S., & Hayden, D. (1990). *Negotiating the special education maze: A guide for parents and teachers*. (2nd Ed.). Rockville,MD: Woodbine House.

Baker, B.L., Brightman, A.J., Blacher, J.B., Heifetz, L.J., Hinshaw, S.P., & Murphy, D.M. (1989). *Steps to independence: A skills training guide for parents and teachers of children with special needs*. (2nd ed.). Baltimore: Paul H. Brookes.

Batshaw, M.L., & Perret, Y.M. (1992). *Children with handicaps: A medical primer*. (3rd ed.). Baltimore: Paul H. Brookes.

Brightman, A.J. (Ed.). (1984). *Ordinary moments: The disabled experience*. Baltimore: University Park Press.

Budoff, M., & Orenstein, A. (1982). *Due process in special education: On going to a hearing*. Cambridge, Mass.: Brookline Books.

Caldwell, B., & Stedman, D. (Eds.). (1977). *Infant education: A guide for helping handicapped children in the first three years*. New York: Walker.

Cougan, T., & Isbell, L. (1983). *We have been there: Families share the joy and struggle of living with mental retardation*. Nashville: Abingdon Press.

Cunningham, C. (1988). *Down Syndrome: An introduction for parents*. Cambridge, MA:Brookline Books.

Dickman, I., & Gordon, S. (1985). *One miracle at a time: How to get help for your disabled child — From the experience of other parents*. New York: Simon & Schuster.

Donnellan, A.M., LaVigna, G.W., Negri-Shoultz, N., & Fassbender L. (1988). *Progress without punishment*. New York: Teachers College Press.

Dougan, T., Isbell, L., & Vyas, P. (1979). *We have been there: A guidebook for families of people with mental retardation.* Nashville: Abingdon Press.

Downs-Taylor, C., & Landon, E.M. (1981). *Collaboration in special education: Children, parents, teachers, and the IEP.* Belmont, CA: Fearon Education.

Duffy, S., McGlynn, K., Manska, J., & Murphy, J. *Acceptance is only the first battle: How some parents of young handicapped children have coped with common problems.* Missoula, MY: Montana University Affiliated Program.

Epilepsy Foundation of America. (1983). *Epilepsy: You and your child, a guide for parents.* Landover, MD: Epilepsy Foundation of America.

Featherstone, H. (1982). *A difference in the family: Life with a disabled child.* New York: Penguin.

Fewell, R., & Vadasy, P. (Eds.). (1986). *Families of handicapped children: Needs and supports across the life span.* Austin: Pro-Ed.

Freeman, R., Carbin, C.F., & Boese, R. (1981). *Can't your child hear? A guide for those who care about deaf children.* Baltimore: University Park Press.

Glidden, L.M. (1989). *Parents for children, children for parents: The adoption alternative.* Washington, D.C.: American Association on Mental Retardation.

Goldfarb, L.A., Brotherson, M.J., Summers, J.A., & Turnbull, A. (1986). *Meeting the challenge of disability or chronic illness — A family guide.* Baltimore: Paul H. Brookes.

Good, J.D, & Reis, J.G. (1985). *A special kind of parenting: Meeting the needs of handicapped children.* Franklin Park, Ill.:La Leche League International.

Greenfeld, Josh. (1975). *A child called Noah.* New York: Pocket Books.

Heally, A., Keesee, P.D., & Smith, B.S. (1989). *Early services for children with special needs: Transactions for family support.* Baltimore: Paul H. Brookes.

Jan, J.E., Ziegler, R.G., & Erba, G. (1983). *Does your child have Epilepsy?* Grand Central Station, NY: University Park Press.

Leff, Patricia T. & Walizer, Elaine H., *(1992) Building the Healing Partnership: Parents, Professionals & Children with Chronic Illnesses and Disabilities.* Cambridge, MA: Brookline Books.

Levy, J.M., Levy, P.H., & Nivin, B. (Eds.). (1989). *Strengthening families: New directions in providing services to people with developmental disabilities and their families.* New York: Young Adult Institute Press.

Lindemann, J.E., & Lindemann, S.J. (1988). *Growing up proud: A parents' guide to the Psychological care of children with disabilities.* New York: Warner Books.

Markel, G.P., & Greenbaum, J. (1985). *Parents are to be seen and heard: Assertiveness in educational planning for handicapped children.* Ann Arbor, Mich.: Greenbaum & Markel.

Masse, S., & Masse, R. (1975). *Journey.* New York: Alfred A. Knopf.

Meyer, D.J., Vadasy, P.F., & Fewell, R.R. (1985). *Living with a brother or sister with special needs: A book for sibs.* Seattle: University of Washington Press.

Middleton, A., Attwell, A., & Walsh, G. (1981). *Epilepsy: A handbook for parents, families, teachers, health & social workers.* Boston: Little, Brown, and Co.

Mindel, E., & Vernon, M. (1971). *They grow in silence: The deaf child and his family.* Silver Spring, MD: Nat'l Assoc. of the Deaf.

Mollan, R. (1981). *Yes they can! A handbook for effectively parenting the handicapped.* Buena Park, CA: Reality Productions.

Parent helper -- Handicapped children birth to five. Maryland State Department of Education. 1982. (Order from Superintendent of Documents, U.S. Government Printing Office, Washington, DC 20402.)

Parent resource directory (For parents and professionals caring for children with chronic illness or disabilities). 2nd ed.). January, 1988. (Available from the Association for the Care of Children's Health, 3615 Wisconsin Ave., NW, Washington, DC 20016. Phone 202-244-1801 or 244-8922.)

Parents guide to the development of pre-school handicapped children: Resources and services. October, 1984. No. 84-5. (Available from National Library Service for the Blind and Physically Handicapped, The Library of Congress, Washington, DC 20542.)

Perske, R. (1985) *Hope for the families: New directions for parents of persons with retardation and other disabilities*. Nashville: Abingdon Press.

Powell, T.H., & Ogle, T.F. (1985). *Brothers and sisters: A special part of exceptional families*. Baltimore: Paul H. Brookes Publishers.

Prensky, A., & Palkes, H. (1982). *Care of the neurologically handicapped child*. New York: Oxford University Press.

Pueschel, S. M., Bernier, J.C., & Weidenman, L.E. (1988). *The special child: A source book for parents of children with developmental disabilities*. Baltimore: Paul H. Brookes.

Reisner, H. (Ed.). (1988). *Children with epilepsy: A parent's guide*. Kensington, MD: Woodbine House.

Routberg, M. (1986). *On becoming a special parent: A mini-support group in a book*. Chicago: Parent/Professional Publications.

Schleichkorn, J. (1983). *Coping with cerebral palsy: Answers to questions parents often ask*. Austin: PRO-ED.

Schleifer, M.J., Klein, S.D. (Eds.). (1985). *The disabled child & the family: An exceptional parent reader*. Boston: The Exceptional Parent Press.

Segal, M. (1988). *In time and with love: Caring for the special needs baby*. New York: Newmarket Press.

Selected readings for parents of preschool handicapped children (A bibliography). July, 1986. No. 86-1. (Available from Nat'l Library Service for the Blind and Physically Handicapped, The Library of Congress, Washington, DC 20542.)

Shore, K. (1986). *The special education handbook: A comprehensive guide for parents and educators*. New York: Teachers College Press.

Simons, R. (1987). *After the tears: Parents talk about raising a child with a disability*. Orlando, Fla.: Harcourt Brace Jovanovich.

Smith, S. (1981). *No easy answers -- The learning disabled child*. New York: Bantam Books.

Thompson, C.E. (1986). *Raising a handicapped child: A helpful guide for parents of the physically disabled*. New York: William Morrow and Co.

Tingey-Michaelis, C. (1983). *Handicapped infants and children: A handbook for parents and professionals*. Austin: Pro-Ed.

Turnbull, H.R., & Turnbull, A.P. (1985). *Parents speak out then and now*.(2nd ed.) Columbus: Charles E. Merrill Publishing Co.

Weiner, F. (1986). *No apologies: A guide to living with a disability, written by the real authorities -- People with disabilities, their families, and friends*. New York: St. Martin's.

Wing, L. (1980). *Autistic children: A guide for parents and professionals*. Secaucus, NJ: Citadel Press.

Glossary

Abduction: Movement away from midline.

Achievement Test: A test measuring what a child has learned, often in specific areas or domains.

Acute: An episode, serious event or illness that starts suddenly and lasts a short time.

Adaptive Behavior: Strategies a child has mastered for coping with tasks in the environment.

Adaptive Equipment: Therapeutic aids such as a special seat, spoon, or stander to facilitate correct positioning and movement.

Adduction: Movement toward midline.

Age Appropriate: Activities and materials are age appropriate when children who are the same age as your child (but who do not have a disability) would typically engage in the activity or use the materials.

Age Equivalent: A test score, expressed in terms of the chronological age at which most children achieve this task or pass this item.

Aggression: Physical or verbal action that causes discomfort or damage to some person or object.

Acquired Immune Deficiency Syndrome (AIDS): This is a serious and potentially fatal disease in which the immune system is no longer able to protect the body and the individual becomes easily ill over a period of years with infections, cancer or other serious diseases.

Amniocentesis: A medical test which occurs before the baby is born. A sample of the mother's amniotic fluid which surrounds the fetus is withdrawn and analyzed to determine the presence of certain birth defects.

Anoxia: A lack of oxygen to the baby which may lead to brain damage.

Anterior: Front or face side of body.

Apnea: Temporary cessation of breathing.

Apgar Score: Score given at birth to describe an infant's neurological status.

Aptitude Test: A means of measuring a child's ability to learn or perform in one or more areas.

Assessment: The process of obtaining and gathering different kinds of information to provide a suitable educational or therapeutic program. This may include tests, observations of the child and interviews with parents.

Assimilation: A term which some educators and psychologists use to describe how a child learns to understand his or her environment. It refers to the process of incorporating new events and experiences into what the child already knows and understands.

Asthma: A chronic condition in which the tissues of the lungs are inflamed and breathing is difficult, especially following allergic reactions.

Asymmetry: One side is unequal or dissimilar to the other.

Attention Deficit Disorder (ADD): A condition in which a child's ability to organize and attend to the environment is impaired sufficiently to hinder learning and acquisition of social skills. Characteristics includes short attention span, trouble concentrating, distractibility, difficulty following more than one command at a time and not appearing to listen.

Audiologist: A highly trained person able to assess hearing both with and without hearing aids, as well as able to test hearing aids for correct functioning.

Auditory Perception: The ability to obtain meaning from what is heard.

Auditory Stimulation Discrimination: The ability to recognize and separate different sounds.

Augmentative Communication: Aids to communication such as a picture book, computer board and sign language that enable a person who is unable to speak to communicate.

Autism: A severe disability which begins in early childhood (usually within the first three years). Characteristics often include abnormal ways of relating to people, objects, and events, absent or delayed speech and language, difficulty with variation in the environment or routines, unconventional use of toys and objects, repetitive movements such as rocking, head banging, and spinning. There are frequently developmental delays and sometimes unusual developmental patterns.

Basal Score: The point on a test at which all previous items have been passed. The basal score may be given in age-equivalent terms.

Baseline: A record of the child's behavior before beginning an intervention. Educators often compare information about the child's behavior after intervention with the baseline to see if the intervention was effective.

Behavior Disorder (BD): A chronic pattern of behavior that violates the social or cultural norms and expectations and may affect educational performance. This may include difficulties in the following areas: relationships with peers or adults; self-care; or inappropriate behaviors to express feelings.

Behavior Management or Behavior Modification: A strategy designed to help a child change specific behaviors by managing environmental stimuli and environmental consequences.

Bilateral: Involving both sides of the body.

Bradycardia: A slowing of the heartbeat often found in premature infants.

Brainstem Auditory Evoked Response (BAER): A test used to evaluate hearing in infants. Electrodes monitor the child's brain waves in response to different levels and frequency of sounds emitted by the testing apparatus.

Bronchopulmonary Dysplasia: A chronic lung disease sometimes seen in premature infants that sometimes follows respiratory distress syndrome.

Cardiology: A branch of medicine which is concerned with the heart and circulatory system.

Ceiling Age: The level on a test where the child can no longer pass more difficult items.

Central Nervous System (CNS): The brain and spinal cord.

Cerebral Palsy: A disability which results from damage to the central nervous system. It results in disturbances of muscle tone, posture and movement.

Child Life Worker: In a hospital, specialists in child development who intervene to provide therapeutic play and learning activities.

Child Protective Services: Social workers or other professional specialists who investigate allegations and incidents of child abuse or neglect. They may also routinely interview parents after serious accidents or unexplained illnesses.

Chronic: A disease or disability that tends to last a long time or has frequent recurrences.

Cleft Palate: An opening in the upper palate of the mouth which is usually treated with surgery. It may occur alone or in combination with other disabilities.

Cognitive Development: The development of the ability to think logically, remember, reason, and to process information about the environment.

Colostomy: An opening into the large intestine through the abdominal wall allowing waste products to be excreted into a bag.

Communication Book/Communication Board: A book or board with pictures or signs to aid a person who is unable to speak to communicate with others.

Confidentiality: Keeping information private. If someone assures confidentiality, they mean that they will not release the information without your permission.

Congenital Disabilities: A disorder or disability that is present at birth.

Congenital Rubella Syndrome: A condition in which the unborn fetus is exposed to the rubella (German measles) virus in the first trimester of pregnancy. It may result in various disabilities including cerebral palsy, cataracts, sensorineural hearing loss, microcephaly, mental retardation, liver disease or heart defects.

Consent: Agreeing to or giving permission for a certain medical procedure, educational program, or placement or intervention on behalf of a child by that child's legal guardian or surrogate parent.

Contractures: Shortening of muscle fibers which limits movement.

Correlation: A statistical method of measuring the relationship between two variables.

CT Scan (CAT Scan): A medical term that refers to an image of a cross section of a person's body which produces a 3-dimensional picture of the tissue density. CAT scans are often used to obtain specific information for the purpose of diagnosis or to monitor certain medical conditions, especially of the brain.

Cystic Fibrosis: An inherited disease resulting in respiratory problems such as chronic coughing, wheezing, and recurring pneumonia.

Cytomegalovirus (CMV): A virus that can infect the fetus and cause birth defects and/or severe illnesses.

Developmental Age: A measure of development stated as an age equivalent.

Developmental Delay: A rate of development which is behind developmental norms.

Developmental Disability: A disability which begins before eighteen years of age and is expected to continue indefinitely. Examples include mental retardation and cerebral palsy.

Diagnosis: The process of identifying the nature of a condition or problem.

Distal: Furthest from the trunk.

Dorsal: Pertaining to the back or back of a body part.

Dyslexia: The impairment of reading ability.

Echolalia: Repetition or imitation of words without regard to their meaning.

Electroencephalogram (EEG): A graphic recording of the brain's electrical activity. It is often used to diagnose seizures or locate lesions or tumors on the brain.

Electrocardiogram (EKG): A graphic recording of the electrical activity of the heart.

Encephalitis: An infection or inflammation of the brain.

Endotracheal Tube (ET Tube): Tube inserted into the windpipe to allow artificial ventilation.

Epilepsy: A disorder of the central nervous system which is characterized by different types of recurring seizures.

Esophagitis: An irritation or inflammation of the esophagus which leads from the mouth and nasal cavity to the stomach.

Evaluation: Using various forms of assessment procedures to collect reliable and valid information to make decisions about educational programs.

Extension: To straighten the body or part of the body.

Eye-Hand Coordination: Use of the eyes and hands together in movement and manipulation of objects.

Fetal Alcohol Syndrome (FAS): A baby born with physical and mental deficits as a result of maternal drinking during pregnancy. The effects include: growth retardation, facial anomalies and mental retardation.

Fine Motor: The use of smaller and more specialized muscles (eyes, hands).

Flexion: Body or part of body is bent.

Fragile X Syndrome: A condition found in individuals in which there is a defect on the X chromosome. The associated developmental problems can include mental retardation and behavior problems.

Gastro-Esophagal Reflux: A condition that occurs when the valve between the stomach and the esophagus closes only partially and undigested food returns into the esophagus or is vomited.

Gastrostomy: An opening in the abdominal wall allowing an individual to be fed by tube when unable to eat normally.

Gene: The basic unit of inheritance. Genes are carried on chromosomes that determine hereditary characteristics.

Generalization: Taking the skills learned with one person, environment or one set of materials and using them with different people, environments or materials.

Gestational Age: The baby's age based on the number of weeks since conception.

Gross Motor: Large muscle activity; those skills that require the use of the total body. Examples are running and walking.

Hearing Impairment: A loss of hearing usually measured in decibels. It may be caused by permanent structural problems in the ear, or the result of infection or serious illness.

Hemiplegia: Paralysis or weakness involving one side of the body.

Hereditary: Genetic characteristics passed on to children from one or both parents.

High Risk: A higher than average risk of developmental disability or of needing special interventions. Many factors can place children at risk, including low birth weight, prematurity, poor living conditions, and so forth. However, it is important to note that not all children who are at risk have later developmental problems

HIV Positive: A condition in which antibodies to the human immune deficiency virus are present in the body. The condition may potentially develop into AIDS.

Hydrocephalus: Accumulation of excess cerebrospinal fluid in the brain that may result in rapid enlargement of the head.

Hyperactivity: An extremely high activity level. It may also be associated with limited ability to stay with one task, short attention span, and distractibility. It may interfere with school performance and family activities.

Hypertonia: Abnormally high muscle tone. The child may seem very stiff or rigid and may arch back, or have trouble bending or unbending his or her arms or legs.

Hypotonia: Abnormally low muscle tone. The child may have trouble maintaining an erect posture, and may seem to sink into floor or chair.

Imitation: Repeating the same movements, sounds and activities observed of others.

Individual Family Service Plan (IFSP): A written plan designed by parents and staff together to reflect the family's goals for the child and family. It is required in most states for children under three.

Individualized Education Program (IEP): A written statement for a child with a disability that describes his or her education program. It must include stated annual goals, short-term instructional objectives and the special education and related services needed. It is required for children over the age of three.

Integration: Placing children with disabilities in programs which also serve children without disabilities.

Itinerant Teacher: A specially trained teacher who usually travels between different schools or intervention settings where the child with unique educational needs receives his or her educational program.

Language Sample: A way of assessing children's communication skills by analyzing what children say.

Lateral: Related to the side.

Lead Agency: A specific agency designated in each state which oversees services for infants and toddlers.

Least Restrictive Environment: The setting in which a child may optimally learn, and which is most like that of his or her same age peers without disabilities.

Low Birth Weight (LBW): An infant weighing less than 2500 grams at birth.

Mainstreaming: The integration of children with disabilities into settings with children without disabilities.

Magnetic Resonance Imaging (MRI): A diagnostic technique provides information about the tissues and can distinguish diseased from healthy tissue.

Means-end: A term used to describe a child's ability to solve a problem by considering a particular course of action (means) that will bring about a desired outcome (end).

Medically Fragile: An expression describing infants or young children experiencing acute or chronic medical conditions which require frequent or intense medical care.

Medicaid: Insurance providing funds for persons (who qualify based on income) to receive necessary medical care including therapeutic services.

Mental Age (MA): This is similar to developmental age. It is a measure of intellectual ability stated as an age equivalent.

Microcephaly: Small head size which usually indicated a slowdown in the growth of the brain.

Midline: The vertical center line of the body. Examples of midline skills involve bringing hands and toys together at the center of the body.

Milestone: A developmental indication that provides the typical age at which most children without disabilities exhibit a particular skill or behavior.

Modeling: Demonstrating a behavior that you want to be imitated.

Monitor: A machine that may be used to record breathing and heart rates and to sound an alarm if there is an abnormality or cessation in rhythm.

Motor Development: The development of activities or skills that are involved in body movements.

Muscle Tone: The degree of tension in the muscle at rest or during movement. Regulated by the central nervous system.

Nasal-gastric Tube (NG Tube): A tube inserted through the nostril, down the esophagus and into the stomach to allow feeding of a person unable to eat or take fluids normally by mouth.

Negative (In response to a medical test): Indicating the absence of a disease, antibody or condition.

Neonatologist: A physician who focuses on the development and treatment of diseases of newborns.

Neurologist: A physician who specializes in the nervous system and the treatment and diagnosis of its diseases and disorders.

Nonverbal Behavior: Behavior that occurs in the absence of spoken language. Communication occurs through gestures, facial expressions, physical closeness and posture.

Object Permanence: A term used by psychologists and educators to describe a child's ability to understand that objects continue to exist even when they are not visible.

Occupational Therapist: Specialist who focuses on such activities as fine motor skills, feeding skills, adaptation of equipment and daily living skills.

Ophthalmologist: A physician who specializes in the diagnosis and treatment of eye disorders.

Orthopedic: Refers to concerns involving skeletal structure of the body, including bones, muscles and joints.

Petit Mal Seizure: A type of seizure characterized by brief episodes of inattention. The individual may appear to be daydreaming or staring into space. It involves little physical reaction.

Phenylketonuria (PKU): A genetic disorder resulting from a build-up of phenylalanine due to an enzyme deficiency. Can result in mental retardation, hyperactivity and seizures if left untreated. Treatment consists of a carefully controlled diet.

Physical Therapist (PT): A specialist concerned with physical movement and positioning, and development of gross motor skills.

Pincer Grasp: Using the thumb and index or middle finger to pick up a small object.

Positive (In response to a medical test): Indicating the presence of a disease, antibody or condition.

Posterior: Back of the body.

Premature Infant: An infant born prior to the 37th week of gestation.

Prenatal: Before birth.

Primitive Reflexes: A group of reflexes that are present at birth. Over time, these reflexes are integrated into more mature patterns of movement in children without disabilities. Examples include the sucking reflex and the rooting reflex.

Prone: Body is positioned lying face down.

Proximal: Nearest to the trunk.

Reliability: In assessment, the extent to which a test measures the same thing consistently.

Respite: A period of rest or relief.

Reinforcement: A consequence that is given as a result of the child's behavior.

Ritalin: A stimulant medication to control hyperactivity in children.

Rotation: To revolve or turn on an axis.

Screening: An initial measurement used to determine whether potential developmental problems exist and to determine the need for more comprehensive evaluation.

Segregation: The practice of placing children with disabilities in a group setting that only includes other children with disabilities.

Seizure: An excessive periodic discharge of electrical activity in the brain. It may be caused by a very high fever.

Self-Help Skills: The ability to take care of self-care needs such as feeding, dressing and toileting.

Self-Injurious Behavior (SIB): Repetitive, self-stimulating behaviors which are destructive and which the child directs toward him or herself.

Self Stimulatory Behavior: Repetitive motor or posturing behaviors. Examples include body-rocking, hand-flapping, and spinning objects.

Sensory Integration: Coordination of information from all the senses to allow for an appropriate response to the environment.

Severe Disabilities: A person with severe disabilities is someone who needs extensive support throughout their life span in areas such as mobility, communication, learning and self-care problems.

Shunt: A small tube which is surgically inserted to allow excess fluid in the brain cavity to drain harmlessly into the abdomen where it can be easily absorbed. It is commonly used to treat hydrocephalus.

Sickle-Cell Anemia (SCA): An inherited chronic blood disease found chiefly among persons of African-American descent, characterized by an abnormal red blood cell containing a defective form of hemoglobin.

Spasticity (Spastic): (See hypertonia)

Spatial Relations: The ability of a person to understand the position of an object in space in relation to one's self and to other objects.

Spina Bifida: A malformation of the spinal column caused by the failure of the spinal column to close completely in the unborn fetus. It results in paralysis below the lesion and is often associated with hydrocephalus. The individual's intelligence may be normal.

Spinal Meningitis: A severe viral attack on the brain and spinal column tissue that can result in hearing loss, retardation, or death.

Standardized Test: An assessment test for which specific conditions for administration have been established and which has been empirically tested to determine norms and psychometric properties.

Startle Response: A reflexive movement which can be elicited by a surprising event, a loud noise or sudden movement. The child may jerk, blink his or her eyes, or throw out arms and extend fingers.

Supine: Body positioned lying on the back.

Supplemental Security Income (SSI): A program funded as part of social security in order to provide financial support for individuals with physical or mental disabilities who are also in financial need.

Stranger Anxiety: A fear of strangers, places and separation from parents normally expressed by infants in the second half of their first year.

Symmetrical: Both sides of body are the same.

Tactile Defensiveness: Over sensitivity to touch.

Tay Sachs: An inherited disorder found most frequently in those of Ashkenazic Jewish ancestry and marked by an enzyme deficiency. The deficiency causes lipids to build up in nerve and brain cells and results in blindness, mental retardation, neurological deterioration and early death.

Tracheotomy: A surgically created opening directly into the trachea to allow ventilation through a tube when an individual is unable to breathe normally.

Trisomy 13 (Patau's Syndrome): A syndrome caused by the presence of an additional chromosome 13. Its characteristics may include cleft lip and palate, small head size, visual impairment, and mental retardation.

Trisomy 18 (Edward's Syndrome): A syndrome caused by the presence of an additional chromosome 18. Its characteristics include low birth weight, mental retardation, and heart defects.

Trisomy 21 (Down Syndrome): A syndrome caused by an additional 21st chromosome. Its characteristics include flattened facial features, slanted eyes, protruding tongue, hypotonia, heart defects and mental retardation.

Turner's Syndrome: A genetic defect in females caused by the presence of only one X chromosome instead of two. Its characteristics include shortness, heart disease, and a webbed neck.

Ventral: Pertaining to the belly or front of a part.

Weight Bearing: Putting weight on various parts of the body.

Weight Shifting: Putting weight on one part of the body and then moving it to another part (needed for walking, etc.).

For More Information: Suggested Readings

Bailey, D.B. & Wolery, M. (1989). *Assessing infant and preschoolers with handicaps*. Columbus: Merrill Publishing Company.

Batshaw, M.L. & Perret, Y.M. (1992). *Children with handicaps: A medical primer* (third edition). Baltimore: Paul H. Brookes Publishing Co.

Bronicki, G.J. & Turnbull, A.P. (1987). Family-professional interactions. in : *Systematic instruction of persons with severe handicaps*. Snell, M. (Ed.) Columbus: Charles E. Merrill Publishing Company, 9-36.

Brown, F. (1987). Meaningful assessment of people with severe and profound handicaps. In: *Systematic instruction of persons with severe handicaps*, Snell, M. (Ed.) Columbus: Charles E. Merrill Publishing Company, 39-63.

Campbell, P.H. (1987). Programming for students with dysfunction in posture and movement. In: *Systematic instruction of persons with severe handicaps*, Snell, M. (Ed.) Columbus: Charles E. Merrill Publishing Co., 84-100.

Ehrenkranz, R., & Warshaw, J. (1983). In: *Diagnosis and management of respiratory disorders in the newborn*, L. Stern, (Ed.) California: Addison-Wesley Publishing Co., 84-100.

Fallen, N.H. & Umansky, W. (1985). *Young children with special needs*. Columbus, OH: Charles E. Merrill Publishing Co.

Gast, D.L., & Wolery, M. (1987). Severe Maladaptive behaviors. In: *Systematic instruction of persons with severe handicaps*. Snell, M. (Ed.) Columbus: Merrill Publishing Company, 300-332.

Harrison, H. (1983). *The premature baby book.* New York: St. Martins Press.

McCubbin, T. (1987). Routine and emergency medical procedures. In: *Systematic instruction of persons with severe handicaps,* Snell, M. (Ed.) Columbus: Merrill Publishing Company, 152-172.

Musick, J.S. & Householder, J. (1988). *Infant Development: From theory to practice.* Belmont, CA: Wadsworth Publishing Company.

Nilsson, L. (1966). *A child is born.* New York: Delacorte Press.

Orelove, F.P. & Sobsey, D. (1991). *Educating children with multiple disabilities.* Baltimore: Paul H. Brookes Publishing Co.

Raver, S.A. (1991). *Strategies for teaching at-risk and handicapped infants and toddlers: A transdisciplinary approach.* New York: Macmillan Publishing Company.

Simeonsson, R. J. (1986). *Psychological and developmental assessment of special children.* Boston, MA: Allyn and Bacon, Inc.

Snell, M.E., (Ed.) (1987). *Systematic Instruction of persons with severe handicaps.* Columbus: Charles E. Merrill Publishing Company.

Snell, M.E. & Grigg, N.C. (1987). Instructional assessment and curriculum development. In: *Systematic instruction of persons with severe handicaps,* Snell, M. (Ed.) Columbus: Charles E. Merrill Publishing Company, 64-109.

Wolery, M. & Smith, P. (1989). In: *Assessing infants and preschoolers with handicaps.,* Bailey, D.B. & Wolery, M. (Eds.) Columbus: Merrill Publishing Company, 447-477.

National Organizations

Alexander Graham Bell Association for
the Deaf
3417 Volta Place, NW
Washington, DC 20007
202-337-5220

American Academy for Cerebral Palsy
and Developmental Medicine
1910 Byrd Avenue, Suite 118
P.O. Box 11086
Richmond, VA 23230-1086
804-282-0036 (for physician referral)

American Association on Mental
Retardation (AAMR)
1719 Kalorama Road, N.W.
Washington, DC 20009
202-387-1968; 1-800-424-3688

American Cleft Palate Association
331 Salk Hall, University of Pittsburgh
Pittsburgh, PA 15261
412-681-9620

American Council on Rural Special
Education (ACRES)
Western Washington University
359 Miller Hall
Bellingham, WA 98225
206-676-3576

American Foundation for the Blind (AFB)
15 West 16th Street
New York, NY 10011
212-620-2000; 800-232-5463

American Society for Deaf Children
814 Thayer Avenue
Silver Spring, MD 20910
301-585-5400 (V/TDD)

American Speech-Language-Hearing
Association (ASHA)
10801 Rockville Pike
Rockville, MD 20852
301-897-5700 (V/TDD)

Association for Persons with Severe
Handicaps (TASH)
11201 Greenwood Ave. North
Seattle, WA 98133
206-361-8870

The Arc- National Headquarters - A
National Organization on Mental
Retardation
500 East Border Street
Suite 300
Arlington, TX 76010

Association for the Care of Children's
Health (ACCH)
7910 Woodmont Avenue
Bethesda, MD 20814
301-654-6549

Autism Society of America
8601 Georgia Ave.
Suite 503
Silver Spring, MD 20910
301-565-0433

Children's National Medical Center
111 Michigan Avenue, N.W.
Washington, DC 20010
202-745-5000; 202-745-3444 (TDD)

Coalition for the Education and Support
of Attention Deficit Disorder (Co-
ADD)
P.O. Box 242
Osseo, MI 55369
612-425-0423

Collaboration Among Parents and Health
Professionals
National Parent Resource Center (CAPP/
NPRC)
also —Technical Assistance to Parent
Programs (TAPP) Network
Federation for Children with Special
Needs
95 Berkeley Street, Suite 104
Boston, MA 02116
617-482-2915; 800-331-0688

Council for Exceptional Children (CEC)
1920 Association Drive
Reston, VA 22091-1589
703-620-3660; 800-873-8255

Epilepsy Foundation of America (EFA)
4351 Garden City Drive, Suite 406
Landover, MD 20785
301-459-3700; 800-EFA-1000

Especially Grandparents
King Count ARC
2230 Eighth Avenue
Seattle, WA 98121

Families of Spinal Muscular Atrophy
P.O. Box 1465
Highland Park, IL 60035
312-432-5551

Fragile X Foundation, The
P.O. Box 300233
Denver, CO 80203
303-861-6630

International Rett Syndrome Association
8511 Rose Marie Drive
Fort Washington, MD 20744
301-248-7031

Learning Disability Association of
America (LDA)
4156 Library Road
Pittsburgh, PA 15234
412-341-1515; 412-341-8077

March of Dimes Birth Defects
Foundation
1275 Mamaroneck Avenue
White Plains, NY 10605
914-428-7100

Muscular Dystrophy Association (MDA)
810 Seventh Avenue
New York, NY 10019
212-586-0808

Muscular Dystrophy Association, Inc.
5350 Shawnee Road, Suite 335
Alexandria, VA 22312
703-941-3277

National Alliance for the Mentally Ill
(NAMI)
2101 Wilson Blvd., Suite 302
Arlington, VA 22201
703-524-7600

National Association of Protection and
Advocacy Systems (NAPAS)
900 Second Street, NE, Suite 211
Washington, DC 20002
202-408-9514

National Association for Visually
Handicapped
22 W. 21st Street
New York, NY 10010
212-889-3141

National Center for Clinical Infant
Programs
2000 14th Street, North, Suite 380
Arlington, VA 22201
703-528-4300

National Down Syndrome Congress
1800 Dempster Street
Park Ridge, IL 60068-1146
312-823-7550; 800-232-NDSC

National Down Syndrome Society
666 Broadway
New York, NY 10012
212-460-9330; 800-221-4602

National Easter Seal Society
70 East Lake Street
Chicago, IL 60601 312-726-6200; 312-726-4258; 800-221-6827

National Head Injury Foundation, Inc.
333 Turnpike Road
Southborough, MA 01772
508-485-9950; 800-444-6443

National Health Information Center
P.O. Box 1133
Washington, DC 20013-1133
301-565-4167; 800-336-4797

National Information Center for Children
and Youth with Handicaps
(NICHCY)
P.O. Box 1492
Washington, DC 20013
703-893-6061; 800-999-5599

National Information Center on Deafness
(NICD)
800 Florida Avenue, NE
Washington, DC 20002
202-651-5051; 202-651-5052 (TDD)

National Institute of Neurological
Disorders and Stroke (NINDS)
National Institutes of Health
U.S. Department of Health and Human
Services
Building 31, Room 8A-16
Bethesda, MD 20892
301-496-5751

National Multiple Sclerosis Society
733 Third Avenue, 6th Floor
New York, NY 10017
212-986-3240

National Organization for Rare Disorders
(NORD)
P.O. Box 8923
New Fairfield, CT 06812
203-746-6518; 800-999-NORD

National Parent Network on Disabilities
1600 Prince Street
Suite 115
Alexandria, Virginia 22314
703-684-6763

National Rehabilitation Information
Center (NARIC)
8455 Colesville Road, Suite 935
Silver Spring, MD 20910-3319
301-588-9284; 800-346-2742

National Spinal Cord Injury Association
600 West Cummings Park, Suite 2000
Woburn, MA 01801
617-935-2722; 800-962-9629

National Sudden Infant Death Syndrome
Foundation
10500 Little Patuxent Parkway, Suite 420
Columbia, MD 21044
800-221-5105

Orton Dyslexia Society
724 York Road
Baltimore, MD 21204
301-296-0232; 800-222-3123

Sibling Information Network
CT University Affiliated Program
991 Main Street, Suite 3A
East Hartford, CT 06108
203-282-7050

Siblings for Significant Change
105 East 22nd Street
New York, NY 10017
212-420-0430

Sick Kids (need) Involved People (SKIP)
990 2nd Avenue, 2nd Floor
New York, NY 10022
212-421-9160; 212-421-9161

Special Needs Adoption Initiative
Office of Human Development Services
Box 1182
Washington, DC 20013

Special Olympics International
1350 New York Avenue NW, Suite 500
Washington, DC 20005-4709, 202-628-
    3630

Spina Bifida Association of America
4590 MacArthur Boulevard, NW
Washington, DC 20007
202-944-3285; 800-621-3141

Spina Bifida Hotline
4590 MacArthur Boulevard, NW
Washington, DC 20007
800-621-3141

Trace Research & Development Center
    on Communication, Control, and
    Computer Access for Handicapped
    Individuals
S-151 Waisman Center, 1500 Highland
    Ave.
University of Wisconsin-Madison
Madison, WI 53705
608-262-6966

United Cerebral Palsy Association, Inc.
1522 K St., NW, Suite 1112
Washington, DC 20005
202-842-1266; 800-872-5827

Williams Syndrome Association
P.O. Box 178373
San Diego, CA 92117-0910
713-376-7072

State Organizations

ALABAMA

Infant/Toddler Contact

Early Intervention Program
Division of Rehabilitation Services
2129 E. South Boulevard
Montgomery, AL 36130-0586
205-281-1973

3-5 Year Old Contact

Division of Special Education and Services
50 North Ripley Street
Montgomery, AL 36130-3901
205-242-8114

Alabama Disabilities Advocacy Program
P.O. Box 870395
Tuscaloosa, AL 35487-0395
205-348-4928

Association for Retarded Citizens/
Alabama
444 South Decatur
Montgomery, AL 36104
205-262-7688

Department of Mental Health and
Mental Retardation
200 Interstate Park Drive, Box 3710
Montgomery , AL 36193-5001
205-271-9208

Division of Special Education Services
State Department of Education
3346 Gordon Persons Building
50 N. Ripley Street

Montgomery, AL 36130-3901
205-242-8114

Early Intervention Program
Division of Rehabilitation, CCS,
Department of Education
2129 East South Blvd.
Montgomery, AL 36111
205-281-8780

Special Education Action Committee
(SEAC)
P.O. Box 161274
Mobile, AL
36616-2274
205-478-1208; 800-222-7322 (In AL)

ALASKA

Infant/Toddler Contact

Department of Health and Social Services
1231 Gambell Street
Anchorage, AK 99811-4627
907-274-1651

3-5 Year Old Contact

Office of Special Services and
Supplemental Programs
State Department of Education
P.O. Box F
Juneau, AK 99811
907-465-2970

Advocacy Services of Alaska
615 East 82nd, Suite 101
Anchorage, AK 99518
907-344-1002

Alaska P.A.R.E.N.T.S.
Resource Center
P.O. Box 32198
Juneau, AK 99803
907-790-2246
800-476-7678 (in AK)

Association for Retarded Citizens/
    Alaska
2211-A Arca Drive
Anchorage, AK 99506
907-277-6677

Division of Mental Health/
    Developmental Disabilities
Department of Health and Social Services
Pouch H-04
Juneau, AK 99811
907-465-3372

Maternal, Child and Family Health
Department of Health & Social Services
1231 Gambell Street, Room 314
Anchorage, AK 99501-4627
907-274-7626

Special Education Parent Team (SEPT)
210 Ferry Way, Suite 200
Juneau, AK 99801
907-586-6806

ARIZONA

Infant/Toddler Contact

1717 West Jefferson Street
Arizona Department of Economic
    Security
Interagency Coordinating Council for
    Infants and Toddlers
P.O. Box 6123, Site Code (801-A-G)
Phoenix, AZ 85005
602-542-5577

3-5 Year Old Contact

State Department of Education
1535 West Jefferson
Phoenix, AZ 85007-3280
602-542-3852

Arizona Center for Law in the Public
    Interest
3724 N. Third Street, Suite 300
Phoenix, AZ 85003
602-252-4904

Association for Retarded Citizens/
    Arizona
5610 S. Central Street
Phoenix, AZ 85040
602-243-1787

Division of Behavioral Health Services
Department of Health Services
411 North 24th Street
Phoenix, AZ 85008
602-220-6506

Interagency Coordinating Council for
    Infants & Toddlers
Department of Economic Security (801-
    A-6)
1841 West Buchanan Street
Phoenix, AZ 85005
602-258-0419. Ext. 36

Office of Children's Rehabilitation
    Services
Department of Health
1740 West Adams, Room 205
Phoenix, AZ 85007
602-542-1860

Pilot Parent Partnerships
2150 East Highland Avenue, #105
Phoenix, AZ 85016
602-468-3001

ARKANSAS

Infant/Toddler Contact

Division of Developmental Disabilities
    Services
Department of Human Services
P.O. Box 1437
Little Rock, AR 72203-1437
501-682-8676

3-5 Year Old Contact

Preschool Programs
State Department of Education
#4 Capitol Mall, Room 105-C
Little Rock, AR 72201
501-682-4222

Advocacy Services, Inc.
Evergreen Place, Suite 201
1100 N. University
Little Rock, AR 72207
501-324-9215
800-482-1174

Association for Retarded Citizens/
    Arkansas
Union Station Square, Suite 406
Little Rock, AR 72201
501-375-4464

Arkansas Parent Support and
    Information Network
Arkansas Disability Coalition
10002 West Markham, Suite B-7
Little Rock, AR 72205
501-221-1330

Department of Human Services
Division of Mental Health Services
4313 West Markham Street
Little Rock, AR 72205
501-371-2374

Division of Developmental Disabilities
    Services
Department of Human Services
P.O. Box 1437
Donaghey Plaza, North-5th Floor, Slot
    2520
Little Rock , AR 72203-1437
501-682-8703

FOCUS, Inc.
2917 King Street, Suite C
Jonesboro, AR
501-935-2750
501-221-1330

CALIFORNIA

Infant/Toddler Contact

Community Services Division
Dept. of Developmental Services
P.O. Box 944202
Sacramento, CA 94244-2020
916-654-2773

3-5 Year Old Contact

Infant/Preschool Unit
State Department of Education
721 Capitol Mall
Sacramento, CA 95814
916-654-2777

Association for Retarded Citizens/
    California
120 I Street, 2nd Floor
Sacramento, CA 95814
916-552-6619

California Children's Services
Department of Health
714 P Street, Room 323
Sacramento, CA 95814
916-322-2090

California Protection & Advocacy, Inc.
101 Howe Street, Suite 185N
Sacramento, CA 95825
916-488-9950; 800-776-5746 (In CA)

Department of Mental Health
1600 9th Street
Sacramento, CA 95814
916-323-8173

Disability Rights Education and Defense
    Fund (DREDF)
2212 6th Street
Berkeley, CA 94710
510-644-2555

Early Intervention Program
Dept. of Developmental Services
1600 9th Street, Room #310
P.O. Box 944202
Sacramento, CA 95814
916-324-2090

Matrix
A Parent Network and Resource Center
P.O. Box 6541
San Rafael, California 94903
415-499-3877

Northern California Coalition for Parent
    Training Information (NCC)
Parents Helping Parents
535 Race Street, Suite 220
San Jose, CA 95126
408-288-5010

Team of Advocates for Special Kids
    (TASK)
100 West Cerritos Avenue
Anaheim, CA 92805-6546
714-533-TASK

COLORADO

Infant/Toddler Contact

Special Education Division
State Department of Education
201 East Colfax Street, Room 301
Denver, CO 80203
303-866-6709

3-5 Year Old Contact

Special Education Division
State Department of Education
201 East Colfax Street, Room 301
Denver, CO 80203
303-866-6710

Association for Retarded Citizens /
    Colorado
4155 E. Jewell Avenue, Suite 916
Denver, CO 80222
303-756-7234

Division of Mental Health
Dept. of Institutions
3520 West Oxford Avenue
Denver, CO 80236
303-762-4073

Handicapped Children's Program
Department of Health
4210 East 11th Avenue
Denver, CO 80220
303-331-8404

The Legal Center
455 Sherman Street, Suite 130
Denver, CO 80203
303-722-0300

PEAK Parent Center, Inc.
6055 Lehman Drive, Suite 101
Colorado Springs, CO 80918
719-531-9400; 800-284-0251 (In CO)

CONNECTICUT

Infant/Toddler Contact

Bureau of Curriculum and Professional
    Development
State Department of Education
P.O. Box 2219
Hartford, CT 06145
203-566-5658

3-5 Year Old Contact

Early Childhood Unit
State Department of Education
P.O. Box 2219
Hartford, CT 06145
203-566-5658

Association for Retarded Citizens/
    Connecticut
1030 New Britain Ave., Suite 102B
West Hartford, CT 06110
203-953-8335

Board of Education and Services for the
    Blind
170 Ridge Road
Wethersfield, CT 06109
203-249-8525

Connecticut Parent Advocacy Center
(CPAC)
P.O. Box 579
East Lyme, CT 06333
203-739-3089; 800-445-2722 (In CT)

Department of Children & Youth
Services
170 Sigourny Street
Hartford, CT 06115
203-566-8614

Department of Mental Health
90 Washington Street
Hartford, CT 06106
203-566-3869

Dept. of Mental Retardation
90 Pitkin Street
East Hartford, CT 06108
203-528-7141

Office of Protection & Advocacy for
Handicapped & Developmentally
Disabled Persons
60 Weston Street
Hartford, CT 06120-1551
203-297-4300; 800-842-7303 (In CT)

DELAWARE

Infant/Toddler Contact

Part H Coordinator
Department of Health & Social Services
1901 North Dupont Highway - Main Bldg.
New Castle, DE 19720
302-577-4643

3-5 Year Old Contact

Delaware Early Childhood
Diagnostic & Intervention Center
Lake Forest So. B. Elem.
Mispillian & West Streets
Harrington, DE 19952
302-398-8945

Association for Retarded Citizens/
Delaware
Tower Office Park
240 N. James Street, Suite B2
Wilmington, DE 19804
302-996-9400

Children with Special Health Care Needs
P.O. Box 637
Dover, DE 19903
302-736-4735

Disabilities Law Program
144 East Market Street
Georgetown, DE 19947
302-856-0038

Division for the Visually Impaired
Health & Social Services
305 West Eighth Street
Wilmington, DE 19801
302-571-3570

Parent Information Center of DE, Inc.
(PIC)
700 Barksdale Road, Suite 6
Newark, DE 19711
302-366-0152

DISTRICT OF COLUMBIA

Infant/Toddler Contact

Office of Early Childhood Development
Commission on Social Services
Dept. of Human Services
609 H Street, NE
Washington, DC 20002
202-727-1839

3-5 Year Old Contact

DC Public Schools
Webster Building
10th and H Streets, N.W.
Washington, DC 20001
202-724-4018

Association for Retarded Citizens/
District of Columbia
900 Varnum Street NE
Washington, DC 20017
202-636-2950

COPE
P.O. Box 90498
Washington, D.C. 20090-0498
202-526-6814

DC Commission on Mental Health
Services
Child, Youth Services Administration
1120 19th Street, NW, Suite 700
Washington , DC 20036
202-673-7784

Health Services for Children with Special
Needs
DC General Hospital, Bldg. 10
19th & Massachusetts Avenue, SE
Washington, DC 20003
202-675-5214

Information, Protection & Advocacy
Center for Handicapped Individuals
(IPACHI)
4455 Connecticut Ave., N.W., Suite B100
Washington, DC 20008
202-966-8081

Logan Child Study Center
3rd and G Streets, NE
Washington, DC 20002
202-724-4800

FLORIDA

Infant/Toddler Contact

Pre-K Handicapped Programs
State Department of Education
Winchester A Buillding, Room 202
Tallahassee, FL 32399-0400
904-488-6830

3-5 Year Old Contact

Pre-K Handicapped Program
Florida Education Center Ste. 544C
325 W. Gaines Street
Tallahassee, FL 32399-0400
904-488-6830

Advocacy Center for Persons with
Disabilities
2671 Executive Center West, Suite 100
Tallahassee, FL 32301-5024
904-488-9071

Association for Retarded Citizens/
Florida
411 E. College Avenue
Tallahassee, FL 32301
904-681-1931

Children's Medical Services Programs
Dept. of Health & Rehabilitation Services
1317 Winewood Blvd., Bldg. 5, Room 129
Tallahassee, FL 32399-0700
904-487-2690

Division of Blind Services
Department of Education
2540 Executive Center Circle, West
Tallahassee, FL 32301
904-488-1330

Family Network on Disabilities
1211 Tech Blvd., Suite 105
Tampa, FL 33619-7833
813-623-4088; 800-825-5736

Parent to Parent of Florida, Inc.
3500 East Fletcher Avenue, Suite 225
Tampa, FL 33612
813-974-5001

GEORGIA

Infant/Toddler Contact

Mental Retardation Section
Dept. of Human Resources
Developmental Services Unit

878 Peachtree Street, Suite 310
Atlanta, GA 30309-3999
404-894-7761

3-5 Year Old Contact

State Department of Education
1970 Twin Towers East
205 Butler Street
Atlanta, GA 30334-1601
404-656-2425

Association for Retarded Citizens/
Georgia
1851 Ram Runway, Suite 104
College Park, GA 30337
404-761-3150

Children's Medical Services
Department of Human Resources
2600 Skyland Drive, N.E.
Atlanta, GA 30319
404-320-0547

Division of Mental Health/Mental
Retardation
Department of Human Resources
878 Peachtree Street, N.E., Room 315
Atlanta, GA 30309
404-894-6300

Early Intervention Programs
Division of Mental Health, Mental
Retardation & Substance Abuse
Department of Human Resources
878 Peachtree Street, Suite 310
Atlanta, GA 30309-3999
404-894-6321

Georgia Advocacy Office, Inc.
1708 Peachtree Street, N.W., Suite 505
Atlanta , GA 30309
404-885-1234; 800-282-4538

Parents Educating Parents (PEP)
Georgia ARC
1851 Ram Runway, Suite 104
College Park, GA 30337
404-761-2745

Parent to Parent of Georgia, Inc.
2939 Flowers Road South, Suite 131
Atlanta, GA 30341
404-451-5484

HAWAII

Infant/Toddler Contact

Zero to Three Hawaii
Children with Special Health Needs
Family Health Services Division
Department of Health
1690 Kapiolani Boulevard (Suite 928)
Honolulu, HI 96814
808-957-0066

3-5 Year Old Contact

Special Needs Branch
Department of Education, Box 2360
3430 Leahi Avenue
Honolulu, HI 96815
808-737-3720

Assisting With Appropriate Rights in
Education (AWARE)
200 North Vineyard Blvd., Suite 103
Honolulu, HI 96817
808-536-9684

Association for Retarded Citizens/
Hawaii
3989 Diamond Head Road
Honolulu, HI 96816
808-737-7995

Behavioral Health Services
Division of Mental Health
Department of Health
1250 Punchbowl Street, 2nd Floor
P.O. Box 3378
Honolulu, HI 96801
808-548-3906

Child & Adolescent MH Division
Department of Health
3627 Kilauea Avenue, Suite 101
Honolulu, HI 96816
808-548-3906

Children with Special Health Needs
    Branch
Department of Health
741-A Sunset Avenue
Honolulu, HI 96816
808-732-3197

Protection and Advocacy Agency
1580 Makaloa Street, Suite 1060
Honolulu, HI 96814
808-949-2922

Special Parent Information Network
335 Merchant Street, Room 353
Honolulu, HI 96813
808-548-2648

Zero-to-3 Hawaii Project
Pan Am Building
1600 Kapiolani Blvd., Suite 925
Honolulu, HI 96814
808-957-0066

IDAHO

Infant/Toddler Contact

Bureau of Developmental Disabilities
Division of Community Rehabilitation
Department of Health and Welfare
450 West State Street
Boise, ID 83720
208-334-5523

3-5 Year Old Contact

State Department of Education
Len B. Jordan Building
650 West State Street
Boise, ID 83720-0001
208-334-3940

Bureau of Developmental Disabilities
Department of Health and Welfare
450 West State Street, 7th Floor
Boise, ID 83720
208-334-5531

Bureau of Maternal & Child Health
Department of Health & Welfare, State
    House
Boise, ID 83720
208-334-5965

Commission for the Blind
341 West Washington Street
Boise , ID 83720-0001
208-334-3940

Co-Ad, Inc.
4477 Emerald, Suite B-100
Boise, ID 83706
208-336-5353

Idaho Parents Unlimited, Inc.
Parent Education Resource Center
4696 Overland Road, Suite 478
Boise, ID 83704
208-342-5884

ILLINOIS

Infant/Toddler Contact

Early Childhood Specialist
Early Childhood Unit
State Board of Education
100 North First Street
Springfield, IL 62777
217-524-0203

3-5 Year Old Contact

Department of Special Education
State Board of Education
100 North First street
Springfield, IL 62777-0001
217-524-4835

Association for Retarded Citizens/
    Illinois
Printer's Square
600 S. Federal Street, Suite 303
Chicago, IL 60605
312-922-6932

Designs for Change
220 South State Street
Room 1900
Chicago, IL 60604
312-922-0317

Family Resource Center on Disabilities
(FRCD)
20 East Jackson Boulevard, Room 900
Chicago, Illinois 60604

Protection and Advocacy, Inc.
11 East Adams
Suite 1200
Chicago, IL. 60603
312-341-0022

INDIANA

Infant/Toddler Contact

Division on Developmental Disabilities
Department of Mental Health
117 East Washington Street
Indianapolis, IN 46204-3647
317-232-2429

3-5 Year Old Contact

Division of Special Education
State Department of Education
229 State House
Indianapolis, IN 46204
317-232-0570

Association for Retarded Citizens/
Indiana
22 E. Washington Street, Suite 210
Indianapolis, IN 46204
317-632-4387

Division of Services for Children with
Special Health Care Needs
State Department of Public Welfare
238 South Meridian Street, 5th Floor
Indianapolis, IN 46225
317-232-4283

Indiana Advocacy Services
850 North Meridian Street, Suite 2-C
Indianapolis, IN 46204
317-232-1150;800-622-4845 (In IN)

Indiana Resource Center for Families
with Special Needs
833 Northside Boulevard
Building #1, Rear
South Bend, IN 46617
219-234-7101

Task Force on Education for the
Handicapped, Inc.
833 Northside Blvd., Bldg. #1 REAR
South Bend, IN 46617
219-234-7101; 800-33204422 (In IN)

IOWA

Infant Toddler Contact

113 Education Center
University of Northern Iowa
Cedar Falls, Iowa 50614
319-273-6997

3-5 Year Old Contact

Bureau of Special Education
State Department of Education
Grimes State Office Building
Des Moines, IA 50319-0146
515-281-5294

Association for Retarded Citizens/Iowa
715 East Locust Street
Des Moines, IA 50309
515-283-2358

Division of Mental Health, Mental
Retardation, & Developmental
Disabilities
Department of Human Services
Hoover State Office Building
East 12th & Walnut Streets
Des Moines, IA 50319-0114
515-281-5126

Iowa Child Health Specialty Clinics
University Hospital School, Room 247
Iowa City, IA 52242
319-356-1118

Iowa Exceptional Parents Center (IEPC)
33 North 12th Street, P.O. Box 1151
Fort Dodge, IA 50501
515-576-5870; 800-383-4777

Iowa Protection and Advocacy Service,
    Inc.
3015 Merle Hay Road, Suite 6
Des Moines, IA 50310
515-278-2502

Programs for Infants and Toddlers with
    Disabilities: Birth through 2
133 Education Center
University of Northern Iowa
Cedar Falls, IA 50614
515-281-3299

State Commission for the Blind
524 Fourth Street
Des Moines, IA 50309
515-281-7999

KANSAS

Infant/ Toddler Contact

Crippled and Chronically Ill Children's
    Program
Dept. of Health & Environment
Landon State Office Building
900 S.W. Jackson, Room 905
Topeka, KS 66620-0001
913-296-6136

3-5 Year Old Contact

Special Education Administration
State Department of Education
120 East 10th Street
Topeka, KS 66612
913-296-3869

Association for Retarded Citizens/
    Kansas
P.O. Box 676
Hays, KS 67601

Child & Adolescent Mental Health
    Programs
SRS/MH & RS
506 North Docking State Office Bldg.
Topeka, KS 66612
913-296-1808

Council on Early Childhood
    Developmental Services
Department of Health & Environment
Landon State Office Bldg.
900 S.W. Jackson, 9th Floor
Topeka, KS 66601
913-296-1329

Families Together, Inc.
1023 S.W. Gage Street
Topeka , KS 66604
913-273-6343

Kansas Advocacy & Protective Services
513 Leavenworth Street, Suite 2
Manhattan, KS 66502
913-776-1541; 800-432-8276

KENTUCKY

Infant/Toddler Contact

Division of Mental Retardation
275 East Main Street
Frankfort, KY 40621
502-564-3844

3-5 Year Old Contact

Office of Exceptional Children
Capitol Plaza Tower, 8th Floor
Frankfort, KY 40601
502-564-4970

Association for Retarded Citizens/
  Kentucky
833 East Main
Frankfort, KY 40601
502-875-5225

Commission for Handicapped Children
Bureau for Human Resources
Department of Human Resources
1405 East Burnett Avenue
Louisville, KY 40217
502-588-4459

Department for the Blind
427 Versailles Road
Frankfort, KY 40601
502-564-4754

Department for Mental Health/Mental
  Retardation Services
Cabinet for Human Resources
275 East Main Street
Frankfort, KY 40601
502-564-4527

Kentucky Special Parent Involvement
  Network (KY-SPIN)
318 West Kentucky Street
Louisville KY 40203
502-589-5717; 584-1104; 800-525-7746

Office for Public Advocacy
Division for Protection and Advocacy
Perimeter Park West
1264 Louisville Road
Frankfort, KY 40601
502-564-2967; 800-372-2988 (In KY)

LOUISIANA

Infant/Toddler Contact

Office of Special Education Services
State Department of Education
P.O. Box 94064
Baton Rouge, LA 70804-9064
504-342-1837

3-5 Year Old Contact

Program Manager - Preschool Programs
Office of Special Education Services
State Department of Education
P.O. Box 94064
Baton Rouge, LA 70804-9064
504-342-1837

Advocacy Center for the Elderly and
  Disabled
210 O'Keefe
Suite 700
New Orleans, LA 70112
504-522-2337; 800-662-7705 (in LA)

Association for Retarded Citizens/
  Louisiana
721 Government St., Suite 102
Baton Rouge, LA 70802
504-383-0742

Division of Blind Services
Office of Human Development
1755 Florida Blvd., P.O. Box 28
Baton Rouge, LA 70821
504-342-5282

Handicapped Children's Services
Office of Preventive & Public Health
  Services
Department of Health & Human
  Resources
P.O. Box 60630
New Orleans, LA 70160
504-568-5070

Office of Human Services
Department of Health & Human
  Resources
P.O. Box 2790
Baton Rouge, LA 70821-2790
504-342-6717

Parent Linc
200 Henry Clay Avenue
New Orleans, LA 70118
504-896-9268

Project PROMPT
1500 Edwards Avenue, Suite 0
Harahan, LA 70123
504-734-7736; 800-766-7736 (in LA)

MAINE

Infant/Toddler Contact

Child Development Services
State House, Station 146
Augusta, ME 04333
207-287-3272

3-5 Year Old Contact

Child Development Services
State House Station 146
Augusta, ME 04333
207-287-3272

Department of Mental Health & Mental
    Retardation
411 State Office Bldg., Station 40
Augusta, ME 04333
207-289-4223

Interagency Coordinating Council Child
    Development Services
87 Winthrop Street
State House, Station #146
Augusta, ME 04333
207-289-3272

Maine Advocacy Services
1 Grand View Place, Suite 1, Box 445
Winthrop, ME 04364
207-377-6202; 800-452-1948 (In ME)

Services for Handicapped Children
Department of Human Services
150 Capitol Street, State House-Station 11
Augusta, ME 04333
207-289-3311

Special Needs Parent Information
    Network (SPIN)
P.O. Box 2067
Augusta, ME 04338-20670
207-582-2504; 800-325-0220 (In ME)

MARYLAND

Infant/Toddler Contact

Program Director, Part H
MD Infant and Toddler Program
One Market Center, Suite 304
300 W. Lexington St., Box 15
Baltimore, MD 21201
410-333-8100

3-5 Year Old Contact

Program Development and Assistance
    Branch
Maryland State Department of Education
200 West Baltimore Street
Baltimore, MD 21201
410-333-2495

Association for Retarded Citizens/
    Maryland
6810 Deerpath Rd., Suite 310
Baltimore, MD 21227
410-379-0400

Division of Child & Adolescent Services
    Unit
Mental Hygiene Administration
Department of Health & Mental Hygiene
201 West Preston Street
Baltimore, MD 21201
410-225-6649

Information & Referral Specialist
MD State Department of Education
200 West Baltimore Street
Baltimore, MD 21201
410-333-2478

Maryland Disability Law Center
2510 St. Paul Street
Baltimore, MD 21202
410-333-7600; 800-233-7201

Make-A-Wish Foundation of Greater
    Washington
Camalier Building
10215 Fernwood Rd., Suite 400A
Bethesda, MD 20817
301-493-6777

Parents Place of Maryland, Inc.
7257 Parkway Drive, Suite 210
Hanover, MD 21076
410-712-0900

Parent Support Network
Infants and Toddlers Program
One Market Center, Suite 304
300 West Lexington St., Box 15
Baltimore, MD 21201
410-333-8100

Project Assist
Department of Special Education
University of Maryland
College Park, MD 20742
301-405-6476

MASSACHUSETTS

Infant/Toddler Contact

Director, Early Childhood
Developmental Services Unit
Division of Family Health Services
Department of Public Health
150 Tremont Street
Boston, MA 02111
617-727-5089

3-5 Year Old Contact

Division of Special Education
State Department of Education
1385 Hancock Street, 3rd Floor
Quincy, MA 02169-5183
617-770-7468

Association for Retarded Citizens/
   Massachusetts
217 South Street
Waltham, MA 02145
617-891-6270

Commission for the Blind
88 Kingston Street
Boston, MA 02111
617-727-5550

Department of Mental Health
24 Farnsworth Street
Boston, MA 02210
617-727-5600

Department of Mental Retardation
160 North Washington Street
Boston, MA 02114
617-727-5608

Disability Law Center, Inc.
11 Beacon Street, Suite 925
Boston, MA 02100
617-723-8455

Division of Early Childhood
Department of Public Health
150 Tremont Street, 2nd Floor
Boston, MA 02111
617-727-5090

Federation for Children with Special
   Needs
95 Berkeley Street
Boston, MA 02116
617-482-2915; 800-331-0688 (in MA)

Office of Children with Special Health
   Care Needs
Department of Public Health
150 Tremont Street
Boston, MA 02111
617-727-5812

MICHIGAN

Infant/Toddler Contact

Early Childhood Education
State Department of Education
P.O.Box 30008
608 West Allegan Street
Lansing, MI 48909
517-373-8483

3-5 Year Old Contact

State Department of Education
P.O. Box 30008
Lansing, MI 48909
517-373-8483

Association for Retarded Citizens/
    Michigan
333 S. Washington Square
Suite 200
Lansing, MI 48933
517-487-5426

Citizens Alliance to Uphold Special
    Education (CAUSE)
313 South Washington Square, Suite LL
Lansing, MI 48933
517-485-4084; 800-221-9105 (In MI)

Commission for the Blind
Department of Labor
309 North Washington Square
P.O. Box 30015
Lansing, MI 48909
517-373-2062

Department of Mental Health
Lewis-Cass Building
320 Walnut Blvd.
Lansing, MI 48926
517-373-3500

Division of Children's Services
Department of Mental Health
320 Walnut Blvd.
Lansing, MI 48913
517-373-0451

Division of Services to Crippled Children
Bureau of Community Services
Department of Public Health
3424 North Logan Street
P.O. Box 30195
Lansing, MI 48909
517-335-8961

Michigan Protection and Advocacy
    Service
106 West Allegan, Suite 210

Lansing, MI 48933
517-487-1755

Parents are Experts: Parents Training
    Parents Project
UCP of Metropolitan Detroit
23677 Greenfield Road
Suite 205
Southfield, MI 48075
313-557-5070

Peer Support Project
530 West Ionia Street, Suite C
Lansing, MI 48933
517-487-9260

MINNESOTA

Infant/Toddler Contact

Interagency Planning Project for Young
    Children with Handicaps
835 Capitol Square Building
550 Cedar Street
St. Paul, MN 55101
612-296-7032

3-5 Year Old Contact

Unique Learner Needs Section
Department of Education
Capitol Square Building, Rm. 812
550 Cedar Street
St. Paul, MN 55101
612-296-7032

Association for Retarded Citizens/
    Minnesota
3225 Lyndale Avenue S.
Minneapolis
MN, MN 55408
612-827-5641

Division of Maternal & Child Health
Department of Health
717 Delaware Street, SE
Minneapolis, MN 55440
612-623-5166

Minnesota Disability Law Center
430 First Avenue, Suite 300
Minneapolis, MN 55401
612-332-1441

Mental Health Division
Dept. of Human Services
Human Services Bldg.
444 Lafayette Road
St. Paul, MN 55155-3825
612-297-0307

PACER Center, Inc.
4826 Chicago Avenue South
Minneapolis, MN 55417
612-827-2966; 800-53-PACER (in MN)

Pilot Parents
201 Ordean Bldg.
Duluth, MN 55802
218-726-4745

State Services for the Blind & Visually
    Handicapped
Department of Jobs and Training
1745 University Avenue
St. Paul, MN 55104
612-642-0508

MISSISSIPPI

Infant/Toddler Contact

Children's Medical Programs
State Board of Health
P.O.Box 1700
2423 North State Street
Jackson, MS 39215-1700
601-960-7427

3-5 Year Old Contact

Mississippi State Department of
    Education
P.O. Box 771 - Sillers Building
Jackson, MS 39205
601-359-3498

Association for Retarded Citizens/
    Mississippi
2727 Old Canton Rd., Suite 173
Jackson, MS 39216
601-362-1830

Association of Developmental
    Organizations of Mississippi
    (ADOM)
332 New Market Drive
Jackson, MS 39209
601-922-3210; 800-231-3721 (in MS)

Children's Medical Program
Department of Health
P.O. Box 1700
Jackson, MS 39215
601-960-7613

Department of Mental Health
1101 Robert E. Lee Bldg.
239 North Lamar Street
Jackson, MS 39201
601-359-1288

Mississippi Protection & Advocacy
    System for Developmental
    Disabilities, Inc.
5330 Executive Place, Suite A
Jackson, MS 39206
601-981-8207

Mississippi Parent Network
425 Louisa Street
Pearl, MS 39208
601-932-7743

MISSOURI

Infant/Toddler Contact

Section of Early Childhood Special
    Education
Department of Elementary and
    Secondary Education
P.O.Box 480
Jefferson City, MO 65102
314-751-0187

3-5 Year Old Contact

Section of Early Childhood Special
    Education
Department of Elementary and
    Secondary Education
P.O.Box 480
Jefferson City, MO 65102
314-751-0187

Coordinator of Special Education
Dept. of Elementary and Secondary
    Education
P.O. Box 480
Jefferson City, MO 65102
314-751-2965

Department of Mental Health
P.O. Box 687
1915 Southridge Drive
Jefferson City, MO 65102
314-751-4122

Missouri Protection & Advocacy Service
925 South Country Club Drive, Unit B-1
Jefferson City, MO 65109
314-893-3333; 800-392-8667 (In MO)

Services for the Blind
Division of Family Services
Department of Social Services
Broadway State Office Bldg.
619 East Capital Avenue
Jefferson City. MO 65101
314-751-4249

Special Health Care Needs
Department of Health
P.O. Box 570
1730 East Elm
Jefferson City, MO 65102
314-751-6246

Missouri Parents Act-IMPACT
1722 W South Glenstone, Suite 125
Springfield, MO 65804
417-882-7434; 800-666-7228 (In MO)

MONTANA

Infant/Toddler Contact

Management Operations Bureau
Developmental Disabilities Division
Department of Social and Rehabilitation
    Services
P.O.Box 4210
Helena, MT 59604
406-444-2995

3-5 Year Old Contact

Management Operations Bureau
Developmental Disabilities Division
Department of Social and Rehabilitation
    Services
P.O.Box 4210
Helena, MT 59604
406-444-2995

Association for Retarded Citizens/
    Montana
7 Willowbend Drive
Billings, MT 59102
406-656-9549

Department of Education Services
Office of Public Instruction
State Capitol
Helena, MT 59602

Mental Health Bureau
Department of Institutions
1539 Eleventh Avenue
Helena, MT 59620
406-444-4902

Montana Advocacy Program
1410 8th Avenue
Helena, MT 59601
406-444-3889; 800-245-4743

Parents, Let's Unite for Kids (PLUK)
EMC/SPED Building, Room 267
1500 North 30th Street
Billings, Mt 59101-0298
406-657-2055

NEBRASKA

Infant/Toddler Contact

Special Education Office
State Department of Education
P.O. Box 94987
301 Centennial Mall South
Lincoln, NE 68509
402-471-2471

3-5 Year Old Contact

Special Education Office
State Department of Education
P.O. Box 94987
301 Centennial Mall South
Lincoln, NE 68509
402-471-2471

Association for Retarded Citizens/
    Nebraska
521 South 14th Street, Suite 211
Lincoln, NE 68508
402-475-4407

Division of Rehabilitation Services for the
    Visually Impaired
Department of Public Institutions
4600 Valley Road
Lincoln, NE 68510
402-471-2891

Medically Handicapped Children's
    Programs
Department of Social Services
301 Centennial Mall South, 5th Floor
Lincoln, NE 68509
402-471-9283

Nebraska Advocacy Services, Inc.
522 Lincoln Center Bldg.
215 Centennial Mall South
Lincoln, NE 68508
402-474-3183

Nebraska Parent's Information &
    Training Center
3610 Dodge Street

Omaha, NE 68131
402-346-0525

Office of Mental Retardation
Department of Public Institutions
P.O. Box 94728
Lincoln, NE 68509
402-471-2851

NEVADA

Infant/Toddler Contact

Department of Human Resources
505 East King Street
Carson City, NV 89701
702-688-2284

3-5 Year Old Contact

Special Education Branch
State Department of Education
Capitol Complex
400 West King Street
Carson City, NV 89710
702-687-3140

Association for Retarded Citizens/
    Nevada
680 South Bailey Street
Fallon, NV 89406
702-423-4760

Nevada Mental Health Institute
Department of Human Resources
480 Galletti Way
Sparks, NV 89431
702-789-0284

Northern Nevada Child & Adolescent
    Mental Health Programs
Child & Adolescent Services
2655 Enterprise Road
Reno, NV 89512
702-789-0300

NTC Parent Connection
2860 E. Flamingo, Suite A
Las Vegas, NV 89121-2922
702-735-2922

Office of Protection & Advocacy, Inc.
2105 Capurro Way, Suite B
Sparks, NV 89431
702-688-1233; 800-992-5715 (In NV)

Project ASSIST;A Direction of Service
    Nevada CHANCE Parent Project
P.O. Box 70247
Reno, NV 89570-0247
702-747-0669; 702-486-6262; 800-522-0066

NEW HAMPSHIRE

Infant/Toddler Contact

Office of Special Education
State Department of Education
105 Pleasant Street
State Office Park, South
Concord, NH 03301
603-271-3741

3-5 Year Old Contact

Office of Special Education
State Department of Education
105 Pleasant Street
State Office Park, South
Concord, NH 03301
603-271-3741

Association for Retarded Citizens/New
    Hampshire
Box 4, 10 Ferry St., Concord Center
Concord, NH 03301
603-228-9092

Bureau of Special Medical Services
Division of Public Health
6 Hazen Drive
Concord, NH
03301-6527
603-271-4596

Disabilities Rights Center
P.O. Box 19
Concord, NH 03302-0019
603-228-0432

Division of Mental Health and
    Developmental Services
State Office Park, South
105 Pleasant Street
Concord, NH 03301
603-271-5013

Parent Information Center (PIC)
151A Manchester Street; P.O. Box 1422
Concord, NH 03302-1422
603-224-7005/224-6299

Special Education Bureau
Department of Education
101 Pleasant Street
Concord, NH 03301-3860
603-271-3741

NEW JERSEY

Infant/Toddler Contact

Division of Special Education
State Department of Education
225 West State Street, CN 500
Trenton, NJ 08625
609-292-7604

3-5 Year Old Contact

Division of Special Education Bureau of
    Program Review and Approval
225 W. State St.
Trenton, NJ 08625
609-292-4692

Association for Retarded Citizens/New
    Jersey
985 Livingston Avenue
New Brunswick, NJ 08902
201-246-2525

Bureau of Children's Services
Division of Mental Health & Hospitals
Capital Center, CN 727
Trenton, NJ 08625
609-777-0702

Commission for the Blind and Visually
   Handicapped
State Board of Control
Department of Institutions & Agencies
Newark Center Bldg.
1100 Raymond Blvd.
Newark, NJ 07102
201-648-2324

Division of Advocacy for the
   Developmentally Disabled
Department of Public Advocate
Hughes Justice Complex CN 850
Trenton, NJ 08625
609-292-9742; 800-792-8600 (In NJ)

Division of Special Education
Department of Education
225 West State Street, P.O. Box CN 500
Trenton, NJ 08625-0001
609-633-683

Special Child Health Services
Department of Health
363 West State Street CN364
Trenton, NJ 08625
609-292-5676

Statewide Parent Advocacy Network
   (SPAN)
516 North Avenue, East
Westfield, NJ 07090
201-654-7726

NEW MEXICO

Infant/Toddler Contact

Department of Health
Developmental Disabilities Bureau
1190 St. Francis Drive
P.O. Box 06110
Santa Fe, NM 87504-0968
505-827-2573

3-5 Year Old Contact

Department of Education
Special Education Unit
Education Building, SE

Santa Fe, NM 87501-2766
505-827-6541

Association for Retarded Citizens/New
   Mexico
3500-G Comanche NE
Albuquerque, NM 87107
505-883-4630

EPICS Project
P.O. Box 788
Beinaillo, New Mexico 87004
505-867-3396

Parents Reaching Out
1127 University N.E.
Albequerque, NM 87102
505-842-9045; 800-524-5176

Protection and Advocacy Systems, Inc.
1720 Louisiana, N.E.
Suite 204
Albuquerque, NM 87110
505-256-3100; 800-432-4682

NEW YORK

Infant/Toddler Contact

Bureau of Child and Adolescent Health
Department of Health
Corning Tower, Room 208
Empire State Plaza
Albany, NY 12237-0618
518-473-7016

3-5 Year Old Contact

State Education Department
Education of Children with
   Handicapping Conditions
Education Bldg. Annex, Room 1073
Albany, NY 12234-0001
518-474-5548

Advocates for Children of New York
24-16 Bridge Plaza South
Long Island, NY 11101
718-729-8866

Association for Retarded Citizens/New
    York
393 Delaware Avenue
Delmar, NY 12054
518-439-8311

Commission for the Blind and Visually
    Handicapped
Department of Social Services
40 North Pearl Street
Albany, NY 12243
518-473-1801

Family Support Project for the
    Developmentally Disabled
North Central Bronx Hospital
3424 Kossuth Ave., Room 15A10
Bronx, NY 10467
212-519-4796 or 4797

New York Commission on Quality of
    Care for the Mentally Disabled
99 Washington Ave., Suite 1002
Albany, NY 12210
518-473-7378

New York State Office of Mental
    Retardation and Developmental
    Disabilities
44 Holland Avenue
Albany, NY 12229
518-473-1997

Parent Network Center
1443 Main Street
Buffalo, NY 14209
716-885-1004

Resources for Children with Special
    Needs
200 Park Avenue South
Suite 816
New York, New York
212-677-4650

NORTH CAROLINA

Infant/Toddler Contact

Chief of Day Services
Division of Mental Health, Mental
    Retardation and Substance Abuse
    Services
Department of Human Resources
325 North Salisburh Street
Raleigh, NC 27611
919-733-3654

3-5 Year Old Contact

Division of Exceptional Children
State Department of Public Instruction
116 West Edenton Street
Raleigh, NC 27611
27603-1712
919-733-3921

Association for Retarded Citizens/North
    Carolina
16 Rowan St., P.O. Box 20545
Raleigh, NC 27619
919-782-4632

Children and Youth Section
Department of Environment, Health &
    National Resources, Maternal &
    Child Health Division
P.O. Box 27687
1330 St. Mary's Street
Raleigh, NC 27611-7687
919-733-7437

Division of Services for the Blind
Dept. of Human Resources
309 Ashe Avenue
Raleigh, NC 27606
919-733-9822

Exceptional Children's Assistance Center
P.O. Box 16
Davidson, N.C. 28036
704-892-1321

Families First Coalition, Inc.
300 Enola Road
Morgantown, N.C. 28655
704-433-2782

Governor's Advocacy Council for
     Persons with Disabilities
1318 Dale Street, Suite 100
Raleigh, NC 27605
919-733-9250; 800-821-6922

NORTH DAKOTA

Infant/Toddler Contact

Developmental Disabilities Division
Department of Human Services
State Capitol
Bismarck, ND 58505
701-224-2768

3-5 Year Old Contact

Developmental Disabilities Division
Department of Human Services
State Capitol
Bismarck, ND 58505
701-224-2768

Association for Retarded Citizens/North
     Dakota
P.O. Box 2776
417-1/2 E. Broadway, #9
Bismarck, ND 58502-2776
701-223-5349

The North Dakota Protection and
     Advocacy Project
400 East Broadway
Suite 515
Bismark, N.D. 58501
700-224-2922; 800-642-6694

Pathfinder Services of North Dakota, Inc.
Pathfinder Parent Center
16th Street and 2nd Ave., S.W.

Arrowhead Shopping Center
Minot, ND 58701
701-852-9426

OHIO

Infant/Toddler Contact

State Department of Health
Early Intervention Program
131 North High Street
P.O. Box 118
Columbus, OH 43215
614-644-8389

3-5 Year Old Contact

Early Childhood Section
State Department of Education
65 South Front Street, Room 202
Columbus, OH 43266
614-466-0224

Association for Retarded Citizens/Ohio
360 S. Third St., Suite 101
Columbus,OH 43215
614-228-4412

Bureau of Children's Services
Department of Mental Health
30 East Broad Street, Room 1135
Columbus, OH 43215
614-466-1984

Child Advocacy Center
106 Wellington Place
Cincinnatti, OH 45219
513-381-2400

Division of Special Education
State Deptartment of Education
933 High Street
Worthington, OH 43085-4017
614-466-2650

Ohio Coalition for the Education of
    Handicapped Children (OCEHC)
1299 Campbell Road, Suite B
Marion, OH 43302
614-382-5452

Ohio Legal Rights Service
8 East Long Street, 6th Floor
Columbus, OH 43215
614-466-7264; 800-282-9181 (In Ohio)

Training Center
933 High Street, Suite 106
Worthington, OH 43085
614-431-1307

OKLAHOMA

Infant/Toddler Contact

Oklahoma Commission for Child &
    Youth
State Department of Education
Oliver Hodge Memorial Education
 Building, Suite 259
2500 North Lincoln Boulevard
Oklahoma City, OK 73105
405-751-0065

3-5 Year Old Contact

Section for Exceptional Children
State Department of Education
Oliver Hodge Memorial Education
 Building, Suite 259
2500 North Lincoln, Suite 363
Oklahoma City, OK 73105
405-521-3351

Children's Medical Services
Medical Services Division
Department of Human Services
4001 North Lincoln Blvd., 4th Floor
Oklahoma City, OK 73105
405-521-3902

Director of Youth Services
Department of Mental Health
P.O. Box 53277, Capitol Station
Oklahoma City, OK 73152
405-271-7474

Parents Reaching Out in OK (PRO-
    Oklahoma)
1917 South Harvard Avenue
Oklahoma City, OK 73128
405-681-9710; 800-PL94-142 (In OK)

Protection & Advocacy Agency for
    Developmental Disability
4150 East 100th Ave.
Cherokee Building, Suite 210
Tulsa, OK 74146
918-664-5883

Special Education Division
Department of Education
Oliver Hodge Memorial Bldg., Room #215
Oklahoma City, OK 73105-4599
405-521-3351

OREGON

Infant/Toddler Contact

Early Intervention Programs
Department of Education
700 Pringle Parkway, SE
Salem, Oregon 97310-0290
503-373-1484

3-5 Year Old Contact

Early Intervention Programs
Department of Education
700 Pringle Parkway, SE
Salem, Oregon 97310-0290
503-373-1484

Association for Retarded Citizens/Oregon
1745 State Street
Salem, OR 97301
503-581-2726

Children's Development & Rehabilitation
Center
Oregon Health Sciences University
P.O. Box 574
Portland, OR 97207
503-279-8362

Office of Child and Adolescent Mental
Health Services
Mental Health and Developmental
Disability Services Division
2575 Bittern Street, NE
Salem, OR 97310-0520
503-378-8406

Oregon Advocacy Center
625 Board of Trade Bldg.
310 S.W. 4th Avenue, Suite 625
Portland, OR 97204-2309
503-243-2081

Oregon COPE Project (Coalition in
Oregon for Parent Education)
999 Locust Street, NE, Box B
Salem, OR 9730
503-373-7477

State Commission for the Blind
535 S.E. 12th Avenue
Portland, OR 97214
503-238-8380

PENNSYLVANIA

Infant/Toddler Contact

Office of Mental Retardation
P.O. Box 2675
Harrisburg, PA 17105
717-787-3700

3-5 Year Old Contact

Special Education Advisor
State Department of Education
333 Market Street
Harrisburg, PA 17126-0333
717-783-691

Association for Retarded Citizens/
Pennsylvania
123 Forster Place
Harrisburg, PA 17102
717-234-2621

Blindness & Visual Services
Department of Public Welfare
901 North 7th Street/P.O. Box 2675
Harrisburg, PA 17105
717-787-6176

Division of Children's Services
Office of Mental Health
Department of Public Welfare
P.O. Box 2675
Harrisburg, PA 17105
717-772-2764

Mentor Parent Program
Route 257, Salina Road, P.O. Box 718
Seneca, PA 16346
814-676-8615; 800-447-1431

Pennsylvania Protection & Advocacy Inc.
116 Pine Street
Harrisburg, PA 17101
717-236-8110; 800-692-7443 (In PA)

Parents Union for Public Schools
311 South Juniper Street, Suite 602
Philadelphia, PA 19107
215-546-1212

Parent Education Network
333 East 7th Avenue
York, PA 17404
717-845-9722; 800-522-5827 (In PA)

PUERTO RICO

Infant/Toddler Contact

Infants & Toddlers with Handicaps
Program
Department of Health
Call Box 70184
San Juan, PR 00936
809-754-9576

Assistant Secretary of Special Education
Department of Education
P.O. Box 759
Hato Rey, PR 00919-0759
809-764-8059

Asociacion De Padres Pro Bienestar/
Ninos Impedidos de PR, Inc.
Box 21301
Rio Piedras, PR 00928
809-763-4665;765-0345

Maternal & Child Health & Crippled
Children's Programs
Department of Health
Call Box 70184
San Juan, PR 00936
809-763-7104

Planning Research and Special Projects
Ombudsman for the Disabled
P.O. Box 5163
Hato Rey, PR 00919-5163
809-766-2333, 809-766-2388

RHODE ISLAND

Infant/Toddler Contact

Department of Health
Division of Family Health
Room 302 - Cannon Building
3 Capital Hill
Providence, RI 02908
401-456-8379

3-5 Year Old Contact

State Department of Elementary and
Secondary Education
Roger Williams Building, Room 209
22 Hayes Street
Providence, RI 02908
401-277-3505

Association for Retarded Citizens/Rhode
Island
99 Bald Hill Road
Cranston, RI 02920
401-463-9191

Division of Children's Mental Health
Services
Department of Children & Their Families
610 Mt. Pleasant Avenue
Providence, RI 02908
401-457-4701

Interagency Coordinating Council
Department of Special Education
Rhode Island College
600 Mt. Pleasant Avenue
Providence, RI 02908
401-456-8599

Parent Training Specialist
Rhode Island Department of Education
22 Hayes Street, Room 209
Providence, RI 02908
401-277-3505

Rhode Island Protection & Advocacy
System, Inc., (RIPAS)
55 Bradford Street, 2nd Floor
Providence, RI 02903
401-831-3150

Services for the Blind
Dept. of Human Services
46 Aborn Street
Providence, RI 0290
401-277-2300

SOUTH CAROLINA

Infant/Toddler Contact

Division of Children's Health
Department of Health and
Environmental Control
2600 Bull Street
Columbia, SC 29201
803-773-4478

3-5 Year Old Contact

Koger Executive Center
100 Executive Center Drive
Santee Building, Suite 210
Columbia, SC 29210
803-737-8710

Association for Retarded Citizens/South
  Carolina
P.O. Box 2198
Columbia, SC 29221
803-754-4763

Commission for the Blind
1430 Confederate Avenue
Columbia, SC 29201
803-734-7520

Mental Health Youth Services
Dept. of Mental Health
2414 Bull Street, Box 485
Columbia, SC 29202
803-734-7859

Parents Reaching Out to Parents
220 Great North Road
Columbia, SC 29202
803-737-4048

PRO-PARENTS
2712 Middleburg Drive, Suite 102
Columbia, SC 29204
803-779-3859

South Carolina Protection & Advocacy
  System for the Handicapped, Inc.
3710 Landmark Drive, Suite 208
Columbia, SC 29204
803-782-0639; 800-922-5225 (In SC)

SOUTH DAKOTA

Infant/Toddler Contact

Section for Special Education
Division of Education
Department of Education and Cultural
  Affairs
700 Governors Drive
Pierre, SD 57501-3133
605-773-4478

3-5 Year Old Contact

Section for Special Education
Division of Education

Department of Education and Cultural
  Affairs
700 Governors Drive
Pierre, SD 57501-2293
605-773-4329

Association for Retarded Citizens/South
  Dakota
706 N. Euclid, P.O. Box 502
Pierre, SD 57501
605-224-8211

Section for Special Education
Richard F. Kneip Building
700 North Illinois Street
Pierre, SD 57501
605-773-3315

Services to the Visually Impaired
700 North Governors Drive
Pierre, SD 57501
605-773-4644

South Dakota Advocacy Project, Inc.
221 South Central Avenue
Pierre, SD 57501
605-224-8294; 800-658-4782 (In SD)

South Dakota Parent Connection
P.O. Box 84813
Sioux Falls, SD 57118-4813
605-335-8844

TENNESSEE

Infant/Toddler Contact

Office of Special Education
State Department of Education
100 Cordell Hull Building
Nashville, TN 37219
615-741-2851

3-5 Year Old Contact

Office of Special Education
Department of Education
132 Cordell Hull Building
Nashville, TN 37219
615-741-2851

Association for Retarded Citizens/
    Tennessee
1805 Hayes, Suite 100
Nashville, TN 37203
615-327-0294

Crippled Children's Services
Department of Health & Environment
436 6th Avenue North, Room 525
Nashville, TN 37219-5402
615-741-735

Tennessee Protection and Advocacy, Inc.
P.O. Box 121257
Nashville, TN 37212
615-298-1080; 800-342-1660 (In TN)

Office of Children & Adolescent Services
Department of Mental Health & Mental
    Retardation
The Doctor's Building
1706 Church Street
Nashville, TN 37219
615-741-3708

Parents Offering Support to Other
    Parents (POSTOP)
801-A Teaberry Lane
Knoxville, TN 37919
615-691-2418

Support and Training for Exceptional
    Parents (STEP)
1805 Hayes Street, Suite 100
Nashville, TN 37203
615-297-3819

TEXAS

Infant/Toddler Contact

Early Childhood Intervention Program
Department of Health
1100 West 49th Street
Austin, TX 78756
512-458-7446

3-5 Year Old Contact

Special Education Programs
Texas Education Agency
William B. Travis Building, Room 5-120
1701 North Congress Ave.
Austin, TX 78701-2486
512-463-9414

Advocacy, Inc.
7800 Shoal Creek Boulevard, Suite 171-E
Austin, TX 78757
512-454-4816; 800-252-9108

Association for Retarded Citizens/Texas
833 Houston Street
Austin, TX 78756
512-454-6694

Children and Youth/Mental Health
    Services
Department of Mental Health & Mental
    Retardation
P.O. Box 12668, Capitol Station
Austin, TX 78711
512-465-4657

Chronically & Disabled Children's
    Services
Department of Health
1100 West 49th Street
Austin, TX 78756-3199
512-458-7355

State Commission for the Blind
4800 North Lamar, P.O. Box 12866
Austin, TX 78711
512-459-2600

Partners Resource Network
6465 Calder Avenue, Suite 202
Beaumont, TX 77706
409-866-4726; 800-866-4973

Project PODER - Texas Fiesta Education
1226 N.W. 18th St.
San Antonio, TX 78207
512-782-8247

Special Kids, Inc.
P.O. Box 61628
Houston, TX 77208-1628
713-643-9576

UTAH

Infant/Toddler Contact

Family Health Services
Department of Health
288 North 1460 West
Salt Lake City, UT 84116-0700
801-538-6922

3-5 Year Old Contact

Utah State Office of Education
Special Education Department
250 East 500 South
Salt Lake City, UT 84111
801-538-7708

Association for Retarded Citizens/Utah
455 East 400 Street, Suite 300
Salt Lake City, UT 84111
801-364-5060

Children's Health Care Services
Division of Family Health services
Department of Health
288 North 1460 West
Salt Lake City, UT 84116-0650
801-538-6165

Division of Mental Health
Department of Social Services
120 North 200 West, 4th Floor
P.O. Box 45500,
Salt Lake City, UT 84145-0500
801-538-4270

Handicapped Children's Services
State Department of Health
P.O. Box 16650-25 BHCS
Salt Lake City, UT 84116-0650
801-538-6165

Legal Center for People with Disabilities
455 East 400 South, Suite 201
Salt Lake City, UT 84111
801-363-1347; 800-662-9080 (In UT)

Parent to Parent
455 East 400 South, Suite 300
Salt Lake City, UT 84111
801-364-5060; 800-888-4058 (In UT)

Services for the Visually Handicapped
Division of Adult Education & Training
309 East 100 South
Salt Lake City, UT 84111
801-533-939

Special Education
State Office of Education
250 East 500 South
Salt Lake City, UT 84111-3204
801-538-7706

Utah Parent Information Center
2290 East, 4500 South, Suite 110
Salt Lake City, UT 84117
801-272-1051; 800-468-1160 (In UT)

VERMONT

Infant/Toddler Contact

Division of Special Education
120 State Street
State Office Building
Montpelier, VT 05602-2703
802-828-3141

3-5 Year Old Contact

Division of Special Education
120 State Street
State Office Building
Montpelier, VT 05602-2703
802-828-3141

Citizen Advocacy, Inc.
Champlain Mill, Box 37
Winooski, VT 05404
802-655-0329

Department of Mental Health
103 South Main Street
Waterbury, VT 05676
802-241-2604

Division of Services for the Blind and
    Visually Handicapped
Department of Social & Rehabilitation
    Services
103 South Main Street
Waterbury, VT 05676
802-241-2211

Parent to Parent Program
69 Champlain Mill
Winooski, VT 05404
802-655-5290

Services for Handicapped Children
Department of Health
1193 North Ave., P.O. Box 70
Burlington, VT 05402
802-863-7338

Vermont Developmental Disabilities Law
    Project
12 North Street
Burlington, VT 05401
802-863-2881

Vermont Parent Information Center
    Network
Association for Retarded Citizens/
    Vermont
37 Champlain Mill
Winooski, VT 05404
802-655-4016

VIRGINIA

Infant/Toddler Contact

Mental Retardation, Children and Youth
    Services
Department of Mental Health, Mental
    Retardation and Substance Abuse
    Service
P.O. Box 1797
Richmond, VA 23214
804-786-3710

3-5 Year Old Contact

Division of Special Education Programs
State Department of Education
P.O. Box 6Q
Richmond, VA 23216-2060
804-225-2402

Association for Retarded Citizens/
    Virginia
6 North 6th Street
Richmond, VA 23219
804-649-8481

Child & Adolescent Mental Health
Department of Mental Health and
    Mental Retardation
P.O. Box 1797
Richmond, VA 23214
804-786-2991

Department for Rights of the Disabled
101 North 14th Street, 17th Floor
Richmond, VA 23219
804-225-2042; 800-552-3962 (In VA)

Department for the Visually
    Handicapped
397 Azalea Avenue
Richmond, VA 23227
804-371-3144

Division of Children's Specialty Services
Department of Health
Madison Building, 6th Floor
109 Governor Street
Richmond, VA 23219
804-786-3691

Parent Education Advocacy Training
    Center (PEATC)
228 South Pitt Street, Room 300
Alexandria, VA 22314
703-836-2953; 800-869-6782

Parent to Parent of Virginia
Family and Children's Service
1518 Willow Lawn Drive
Richmond, VA 23230
804-282-42551

WASHINGTON

Infant/Toddler Contact

Birth to Six Planning Project
Department of Social & Health Services
P.O. Box 45201
Olympia, WA 98504
206-586-8696

3-5 Year Old Contact

Office of the Superintendent of Public
　Instruction
P.O. Box 47200
Olympia, WA 98504
206-753-0317

Association for Retarded Citizens/
　Washington
1703 East State Street
Olympia, WA 98506
206-357-5596

Children & Adolescent Services
Mental Health Division
Department of Social & Health Services
Mail Stop OB-42F
Olympia, WA 98504
206-753-3900

Parents Advocating Vocational
　Education (PAVE)
6316 South 12th street
Tacoma, WA 98465
206-565-2266; 800-572-7368 (In WA)

PAVE/STOMP - Specialized Training of
　Military Parents
12208 Pacific Highway, SW
Tacoma, WA 98499
206-588-1741

Pierce County Parent to Parent
12208 Pacific Highway, SW
Tacoma, WA 98499
206-588-1741

State Services for the Blind
521 East Legion Way, MS:FD-11

Olympia, WA 98504
206-586-1224

A Touchstone Program
6721 51st Avenue, S.
Seattle, WA 98118
206-721-0867

Washington Protection & Advocacy
　System
1401 East Jefferson
Seattle, WA 98122
206-324-1521

WEST VIRGINIA

Infant/Toddler Contact

Office of Behavioral Health Services
Department of Health & Human Services
1800 Washington Street East
Charleston, WV 25303
304-348-2183

3-5 Year Old Contact

State Department of Education
Office of Special Education Programs
　and Assurances
Building 6, Room B-304, Capitol Complex
1900 Kanawha Boulevard East
Charleston, WV 25305
304-558-2696

Association for Retarded Citizens/West
　Virginia
16 Echo Terrace
Wheeling, WV 26003
304-233-0600

Division of Handicapped Children
Department of Human Services
1116 Quarrier Street
Charleston, WV 25301
304-348-6330

Project STEP
116 East King Street
Martinsburg, WV 25401
304-263-HELP

West Virginia Advocates, Inc.
1524 Kanawha Boulevard, East
Charleston, WV 25311
304-346-0847; 800-950-5250 (In WV)

West Virginia Parent Training and
Information
Schroath Professional Building
2nd Floor, Suite 2-1
229 Washington Ave.
Clarksburg, WV 26301
304-624-1436

WISCONSIN

Infant/Toddler Contact

Bureau of Community Programs
1 West Wilson Street, Room 418
P.O. Box 7850
Madison, WI 53702
608-267-3270

3-5 Year Old Contact

Division for Handicapped Children and
Pupil Services
Department of Public Instruction
P.O. Box 7841
Madison, WI 53707
608-267-9172

Association for Retarded Citizens/
Wisconsin
121 South Hancock Street
Madison, WI 53703
608-251-9272

Bureau for Children with Physical Needs
125 South Webster Street
P.O. Box 7841
Madison, WI 53707
608-266-3886

Office of Mental Health
Department of Health & Social Services
P.O. Box 7851
Madison, WI 53707
608-266-3249

Parent Education Project of Wisconsin,
Inc.
2001 West Vliet St.
Milwaukee, WI 53205
414-937-8380

Wisconsin Coalition for Advocacy
16 North Carroll Street, Suite 400
Madison, WI 53703
608-267-0214

WYOMING

Infant/Toddler Contact

Developmental Disabilities Program
Division of Community Programs
Department of Health and Social Services
354 Hathaway Building
Cheyenne, WY 82002-0710
307-777-5246

3-5 Year Old Contact

State Department of Education
Federal Program Unit
2300 Capitol Avenue
Cheyenne, WY 82002-0050
307-777-7414

Association for Retarded Citizens/
Wyoming
P.O. Box 2161
Casper, WY 82602
307-237-9110

Division of Community Programs
Department of Health & Social Services
356 Hathaway Building
Cheyenne, WY 82002-0710
307-777-7115

Wyoming Parent Information Center
270 Fort Street
Buffalo, Wyoming 82834

Wyoming Protection & Advocacy System
2424 Pioneer Avenue, #101
Cheyenne, WY 82001
307-638-7668; 800-624-7648 (In WY)

Index